Women's, Women's Health

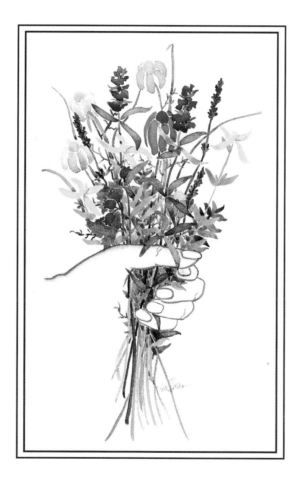

CHRISTOPHER HOBBS, L.AC.
& KATHI KEVILLE

Dedication

In gratitude to my mother, and to my partner Beth, and all the other women whom I've had the pleasure of knowing, and who helped me get in touch with my feminine side.

—Christopher Hobbs

To every woman who opens this book in search of better health and healing. May the knowledge it holds empower your journey.

—Kathi Keville

Acknowledgments

Special thanks to Bill Schoenbart, L.Ac., for writing much of the information on Traditional Chinese Medicine and helping with the osteoporosis and fibroids chapters; and to Stephen Brown, N.D., for his research, insights, and writing on the osteoporosis chapter. We are grateful to Raven Lang, L.Ac., O.M.D., for sharing her many years of experience with pregnancy and birthing. These practitioners and writers made significant contributions to *Women's Herbs, Women's Health*.

We also acknowledge with gratitude all the wise women, midwives, herbalists, and other healers who have added immeasurably to our knowledge of women's health and women's herbs since the beginning.

We thank the editors and artists at Interweave Press who helped make this book a reality.

Disclaimer

Women's Herbs, Women's Health
Christopher Hobbs and Kathi Keville

Cover design: Bren Frisch
Cover painting: Ann Swanson
Illustrations: Susan Strawn Bailey and Gayle Ford
Book design: Dean Howes

Text copyright 1998, Christopher Hobbs and Kathi Keville

Botanica Press is an imprint of Interweave Press

Interweave Press, Inc.
201 East Fourth Street
Loveland, Colorado 80537-5655
USA

Printed in the United States of America

Library of Congress Cataloging-in-Publication Data

Hobbs, Christopher, 1944–
    Women's herbs, women's health / by Christopher Hobbs and Kathi
  Keville.
        p.   cm.
    Includes bibliographical references and index.
    ISBN 1–883010–47–0 (paperback)
    1. Herbs—Therapeutic use. 2. Women—Health and hygiene.
   3. Women—Diseases—Alternative treatments. I. Keville, Kathi.
  RM666.H33H616 1998
  615'.321'082—dc21   98-4414
                                       CIP

First Printing: IWP — 10M:598:Que

FOREWORD

*I*t is an honor and a delight to write a foreword for a work that is not only an impressive contribution to women's search for natural health, but also one written by my favorite herbalists, practitioners I have known for more than twenty years. Christopher Hobbs, Kathi Keville, and I were budding young herb enthusiasts when herbalism in this country was just beginning to rise from its underground status. Today, I consider Christopher my personal "family doctor" and Kathi a source of great inspiration and information.

When they first mentioned they were collaborating on an herb book for women, I responded with enthusiasm. So did others in the ever-growing herbal-health field. I never doubted that Christopher and Kathi would create a refreshing addition to the field of women's health, not just another rehash of information easily found elsewhere.

Women and healing herbs seem to have a remarkable affinity, as witnessed by the number of women who want to learn more about using herbs to treat common health problems. Herbalism itself has long been considered a woman's healing art—not because men aren't excellent herbalists, nor because effective herbal remedies for men don't exist. But herbalism is essentially feminine; it embodies the qualities of intuition, trust, and gentleness, attributes often associated with one's "feminine side." It depends on plants that have evolved over centuries, rooted in the heart of the earth and nourished by the light of the moon.

My highest criterion for a good herb book—especially one about a topic as critical as women's health—is that it be written by a practicing herbalist, someone who knows plants from personal experience. I also look for that nebulous "cellular knowing" that herbalists so often mention, a reference to deep instinctual memories that the plants seem to impart to certain people. *Women's Herbs, Women's Health* exceeds these criteria. Together, Christopher and Kathi have more than sixty years of personal experience using herbs in healing. Christopher's knowledge comes from four generations of family experts. Kathi's love of plants since childhood also reflects this "cellular knowing."

Equal to the authors' personal expertise is the sensitivity, wisdom, and depth of commitment inherent in their work. You'll find it in every page. Easily understood, practical, and rooted in the traditions of herbalism, *Women's Herbs, Women's Health* presents current information, clinical studies, and controversial subjects in an intelligent manner, making it particularly valuable for the contemporary woman. Christopher and Kathi have created a wonderful resource, one that is infused with the history of herbalism and colorfully garnished with the essence of who they are.

—Rosemary Gladstar
East Barre, Vermont

INTRODUCTION

omen's Herbs, Women's Health discusses the major women's health issues of today in a way that is understandable, yet comprehensive. This book is designed to provide you with the tools and answers you need to stay healthy. Whether you are in good or poor health, young or old, natural medicine—and especially herbal medicine—offers time-honored and safe treatments and preventive measures. You will find *Women's Herbs, Women's Health* a sourcebook of knowledge about how your body works, both in medical terms and in the view of traditional medicine. In this book we explore some of the most common reproductive ailments of women. A 1995 review of reproductive-tract disorders resulting in hospitalization in the United States showed that the five most common diseases included pelvic inflammatory disease (49 percent), ovarian cysts (33 percent), endometriosis (32 percent), menstrual disorders (31 percent), and uterine fibroids (30 percent).

To write this book, we have each drawn from our thirty years of clinical and practical experience as holistic practitioners of Western herbal medicine and Traditional Chinese Medicine. We have used what patients, family, and friends have taught us, and have combed the modern medical research thoroughly to address major issues and health questions for women today, including:

- Why is there conflicting information about natural progesterone and estrogen replacement?
- What are the risks of estrogen-replacement therapy?
- How often should I get a Pap smear?
- How can I use herbs to increase wellness and prevent disease?

Such questions are much easier to answer when you are informed about the most current research, remedies, and resources that connect you with other people interested in the same health issues. We hope this book will make a contribution to the empowerment of women and freedom of choice in health care.

This freedom is every woman's right. We will offer our opinions and suggestions, but you are the one who will ultimately make the health decisions about your body. We feel that the more information you have, the better equipped you will be to shoulder this task.

As you take this responsibility, you join the ranks of generations of women who have turned to the gentle healing power of herbs. Although most herb texts since ancient times have been written by men, it is women who have always been the primary caregivers to the sick. The women tended their backyard gardens and used the herbs they grew or gathered from the wild to treat ailments of many types.

The first medical textbook devoted solely to women's health issues was not published until 1995. In this textbook, *The Medical Care of Women*, Suzanne Fletcher, M.D. and her husband write in the introduction, "The relative lack of attention to women's health care in the past probably had several roots. First, with so few women physicians until recently, few physicians, and therefore few educators, writers, and researchers, had firsthand experience with women's health problems. (If men had menses, would male physicians have ever doubted the existence of physical menstrual pain or premenstrual syndrome?)"

By contrast, the practice of herbalism has long given ample attention to women's health issues and diseases. The Eclectic doctors, trained physicians of the early twentieth century who believed in using herbal medicines almost exclusively, focused a good deal of attention on women's complaints. Much of the clinical information about women's herbs originates in the writings of Eclectic doctors.

Even today, most of the students in our classes are women following the age-old tradition of women healers and herbalists. It is likely that you have an ancestor who used herbs for healing. This is the way that herbal knowledge has been passed down for thousands of years. We invite you to join this transmission of knowledge and connection with the healing plants.

You will find that although we have enhanced herbalism with modern viewpoints, physiology, and plant chemistry, it remains a direct form of healing. If you know the plants, you can go out in your backyard or into the woods and collect your own medicine, as people have been doing for thousands of years.

We encourage you to grow herbs in your garden, get to know local wild herbs, eat wild greens, enjoy the taste and aroma of herb tea, and begin to develop a relationship with the healing power of plants. Our knowledge and experience and that of many others show that this practice will not only improve your health but also will enrich your life.

CONTENTS

Chapter 1

WOMEN'S HEALTH

Welcome to the world of natural healing. It is one that we feel certain will improve your life. If you have already used natural remedies, then you personally know how beneficial they can be. If you haven't, we hope you will be encouraged to explore them.

Each chapter of this book focuses on a major condition or body system. You may be inclined to turn to the pages that address a health problem you are currently facing, but we encourage you to take a few minutes to read this chapter first. The information in it will help you better understand the principles of holistic healing and how to apply them to your own natural health plan.

This book goes beyond the use of herbs to encompass natural healing in a broad sense. Although we both use herbs as our primary mode of healing, we find that they often work better when lifestyle changes and other natural healing strategies are incorporated. We give an herbal remedy for each condition, but also explain how to treat it with other methods, including lifestyle and nutritional changes. As health professionals with experience in herbs, acupuncture, massage, and aromatherapy, we heartily recommend these techniques, as well as other types of bodywork, as a part of your health regimen.

Research strongly indicates that for women of any age, a healthy lifestyle is the key to maintaining health. At a November, 1997 conference on aging and health habits, Dr. Edward Schneider, dean of the Gerontology Center at the University of Southern California, said, "Personal choice has more impact on health later in life than genetics." Schneider believes that exercise is the best prescription against aging, because it improves cardiopulmonary fitness, slows osteoporosis, helps ease arthritis, promotes sleep, and simply makes you feel better. Another attendee, Dr. William Haskell, recommended about thirty minutes a day of vigorous physical activity. "No medication, no diet pill, no *ginkgo biloba*," Haskell said, "will replace exercise in maintaining physical functioning." William Evans

California poppy

of the U.S. Department of Agriculture and Human Nutrition Research Center on Aging at Tufts University said, "Much of what we call aging is nothing more than an accumulation of a lifetime of inactivity." Starting in middle age, he said, women start to lose muscle, bone strength, and aerobic capacity—and to gain fat.

Speaking of fat, extra weight is one of the biggest challenges facing women in North America. Being overweight has been linked with an increased risk of developing breast and uterine cancer as well as heart disease and diabetes. A recent population study reported that about 51 percent of all Canadians are either overweight or obese. The World Health Organization has recently reported that the rate of obesity is doubling every five years in many countries. While herbs can be helpful in weight-loss programs, there simply is no substitute for exercise and a healthy diet rich in vegetables and fruits, moderate in protein, and low in fat.

Another important factor in women's health is maintaining warm and frequent contact with friends and family members—in other words, happiness. In one study of 276 women volunteers who were purposely infected with the cold virus, researchers at the University of Pittsburgh School of Medicine discovered that the more social interactions an individual had, the less likely she was to develop a cold. Dr. Bruce Rabin, a spokesperson for the study, said, "The message is clear: loneliness is associated with decreased immune system function."

The next line of defense after diet, lifestyle, and herbs is nutritional supplements. Although minerals, vitamins, and other food-based supplements are isolated and processed, they still offer a relatively natural road to health. Food and nutrient technology has advanced tremendously, and a wide array of concentrated phytonutrients, such as the free-radical fighting oligomeric proanthocyanidins, or OPCs, are available today. Because few of us are able to eat all of the fruits and vegetables we need to get the nutrients for optimum health, we review nutritional supplements that can assist your healing in most of the chapters of this book.

The techniques of modern Western medicine are also available to you. Indeed, without the assistance of the best that medical science has to offer, some of the conditions we discuss in this book would remain undetected until they became life-threatening. In the chapters to come, we'll explain the risks and benefits of these healing strategies, as well as the natural alternatives, so that you can make the best decision for yourself. Our dream is that natural healing will be partnered with modern medicine, and that health-care professionals will use all the appropriate methods to restore their patients to total health.

OUR APPROACH TO HEALING

There are some vast differences between the overall philosophy of Western medicine and the natural healing techniques that we use. This chapter will help you understand these differences. Physicians have been thoroughly trained in the intricate workings of the body. They use sophisticated tests to detect subtle changes in enzyme, hormone, and nutrient levels. They can set bones and remove life-threatening tumors. In the past, however, medical schools have seldom emphasized the role that nutrition and common health practices play. Western medicine tends to focus on disease and how to treat it. Natural medicine, and especially herbal medicine, seeks to understand health and how to create and preserve it throughout life. We hope the preventive medicine strategies in this book help you spend your money on staying healthy instead of spending it on medicine after you are sick.

One fundamental element of this approach is that the relationship between the health-care practitioner and the patient should be a partnership. The doctor brings powers of observation, knowledge, skills, and caring. What you bring to this relationship is as important or more. Your receptivity to new ways, new habits, and your ability to listen closely to the needs of your body and spirit will be crucial to your success in restoring or maintaining your health.

The beauty of herbs is that they work with your body, not on it. Herbal remedies encourage the body to heal itself. When, for example, herbs stimulate the body's defenses to fight a virus or strengthen and cleanse an organ, the body is working with its own resources instead of relying on a substance from outside it. And the healing changes that occur are often longer-lasting, although they also may take longer to occur.

About Constitutional Herbalism

There is much, much more to using herbs than simply substituting a single herb for a particular drug. For one thing, herbalists and other holistic practitioners focus on the cause of a problem, then use herbs and other forms of natural healing to address not only the problem's symptoms, but

---

COMMUNICATION IS THE KEY

We believe that alternative healing methods, including herbal remedies, have much to offer both patients and Western-trained physicians. But one thing is essential: if you are under a doctor's care for a condition, and especially if you are already taking prescription or over-the-counter drugs, communicate with your physician about your intent to try herbal remedies for that condition. Some herbs can have adverse interactions with pharmaceutical drugs; others, such as St. John's wort, can be substituted for pharmaceutical drugs but only carefully and gradually. If your doctor is not open to trying noninvasive, gentle natural remedies before or concurrently with other therapies, we suggest you find a physician who will consider them.

its source. Another benefit to herbalism and other traditional medical systems is that they take into account the individual idiosyncrasies of the patient— physique, level of fitness, the speed and character of the patient's metabolism, lifestyle and work conditions. This blending of modern and traditional Western herbalism with traditional philosophies that emphasize metabolism type is called constitutional herbalism.

To understand the difference between this approach, and that of Western scientific research, consider the following. When scientific researchers study a particular treatment, like a new birth-control pill to relieve symptoms of PMS, they often get mixed results, even though as many study variables as possible are controlled. In some women, the treatment helps relieve many PMS symptoms, such as mood swings, food cravings, bloating, or uterine cramps. In others, the pill offers no relief whatsoever, and in others still, it may exacerbate symptoms. This happens because the women are unique individuals, and their symptoms, though they may be sorted into similar categories, are also unique. Medical research often considers only a disease and the drug that treats it, rather than the individuals affected.

Along with other modern Western herbalists, we have been increasingly influenced by the herbal traditions of other cultures. Traditional Chinese Medicine (TCM) is a system of treatment that has developed over 4,000 years. Ayurveda, the ancient East Indian system of healing, is another tradition that modern herbalists are exploring. Both of these ancient systems emphasize the unique nature of both the patient and the herbal medicines and healing foods. In these systems, health is understood to be created when an individual understands her or his own nature and can eat the foods and embrace the daily habits that can work with that nature instead of against it. For instance, if a woman has a very fast and responsive nervous system that is easily aroused, she can achieve greater health by seeking foods, drinks, and activities that will foster calmness and steadiness. Imagine Karen—a thin, wiry, nervous young woman, always on the go. She is a sales rep for a large manufacturing company. Her job is to visit stores in a large metropolitan area. She is constantly driving in heavy traffic and wooing potential customers. Karen is burning out after two years on the job. Its frenetic nature exhausts her to the point where she reaches for coffee and chocolate to keep going, then alcohol to calm down. The principles of Ayurveda suggest that Karen's ideal foods might include calming grains and beans, vegetables, and fish, with few spicy or concentrated sweet foods. To help repair the damage from the stress of her job, we would recommend calming and sleep-promoting herbs, formulas that support her adrenal glands, and bodywork and exercise that help remove the waste products produced by stress. As you try the herbal and nutritional remedies we recommend in this book, keep in mind your own constitutional nature and individual needs.

Some Important Herbal Concepts

Herbal remedies are allies when it comes to relieving symptoms associated with women's health problems. They can restore balance, make up deficiencies, and reinstate the health and integrity of tissues and organs, including ones that directly affect the menstrual cycle, mood and emotions, the cardiovascular system, and other aspects of your health.

To get the most out of the herbal remedies in this book, or to adapt them for your own needs, you will need to grasp a few concepts about how Western herbalists use herbs.

Tonics

This is a category of herbs that includes nettle leaf, American ginseng root, and many others that generally support the nutrition and repair of the body or a specific organ or system. For example, if your immune system is weak and run-down and you are prone to repeated colds or vaginal yeast infections, tonic herbs for your immune system will help restore its strength and allow it to do its job in eliminating the infections quickly. Tonic herbs are most effective when used in a full course of treatment, meaning the herbs must be taken consistently for a minimum of three months, sometimes as long as a year. The benefits tonic herbs offer can be tremendous if the user is patient and consistent. How long you will need to take tonic herbs depends on the severity of your weakness and how long it has been developing. A professional herbalist can help you determine the best course of treatment with tonic herbs.

Tonic herbs work gently during an acute infection of any kind—a fever or sore throat, for example, or a vaginal yeast infection—so concentrate on taking specific herbs to treat your condition.

TONICS AND SPECIFICS

Some Common Tonic Herbs

Alfalfa

Dong quai

Ginseng

Hawthorn

Horsetail

Milk thistle

Nettles

Red raspberry

Reishi

Siberian ginseng

Wild oats

Some Common Specific Herbs

Black cohosh

Chamomile

Ginkgo

Goldenseal

Lemon balm

Oregon grape root

Partridge berry

Red clover

St. John's wort

Vitex

Specifics

This is the name used for herbs that help a specific organ or system to heal or work more efficiently. These herbs are used for shorter periods of time, because they are essentially stimulants for these organs or systems. Echinacea, for example, is a stimulant for the immune system. It is best taken for several days, just as you feel the first twinge of a cold or yeast infection. It revs up your immune engine to fight the invading virus or microorganism. But just as constantly racing your car's engine increases wear and tear on the system, herbalists don't recommend taking echinacea continually. Nor should you take it if you have a long-standing immune weakness or disorder except under the supervision of an experienced herbal practitioner. That's like racing a car engine that is in disrepair. Instead, take specific herbs for several days to a month or so and then stop. If the problem is not resolved, try another course of the herbs, but be aware that if stimulating herbs are not working, the organs and tissues involved may need more support and healing through the use of tonics for a few months. Tonics and specifics can be used together. For instance, if you suddenly develop a bladder infection, you will want to try an herbal formula with herbs such as uva-ursi, juniper berry, usnea, and barberry to discourage the bacteria and help clear the infection. But if you get repeated bladder infections, even after the use of antibiotics, then a two- or three-month course of bladder tonics, such as goldenrod, pipsissewa, saw palmetto, and nettle root, is in order. During the acute phase of an infection, let the anti-bacterial herbs predominate supported by a few of the tonics. When the infection is waning, focus on the tonic herbs, adding a few soothing herbs, such as marshmallow root and licorice.

SOME COMMON CLEANSING HERBS

Cleansing herbs include:

Burdock root

Psyllium husk and seeds

Red clover

Sarsaparilla

Yellow dock root

Cleansers

This group includes herbs that assist the body by stimulating immune function, increasing elimination through the bowels, skin, and kidneys. Cleansers also help increase the liver's ability to process toxins. Herbalists believe that if you have a skin problem such as acne, boils, or dandruff, increasing elimination of waste products through the bowels and kidneys will help stop it at its source. Herbs that work mainly to clean the blood and circulatory system belong to a particular category of cleansers called "blood purifiers."

How We Use Traditional Chinese Medicine

Traditional Chinese Medicine is rooted in our connection with nature, the seasons, animals, plants, and our own societies. Unlike Western medicine, which seeks to understand the specific cause of a specific disease, TCM tries to comprehend the whole design of life. Environmental conditions such as heat, cold, dampness, and dryness, along with the emotions fear, anger, sadness, worry, and joy, strongly influence health or sickness. The strength of a patient's constitution, inherited from forebears, and her way of life complete the picture.

This system of medicine uses herbs and other remedies not only according to their specific effects on individual symptoms, but as multi-dimensional forces with many useful qualities. These qualities help us decide how and when to apply an herb or food for a particular need. For instance, Traditional Chinese Medicine sees bronchitis as a "hot" infection. In such a case, it is best to use "cool" herbs, such as usnea lichen or barberry, to help reduce the heat and clear the infection. A "warm" herb, such as cinnamon or ginger, could make the condition worse. In Traditional Chinese Medicine, each herb or medicinal food has its own energetic properties, among other qualities. Chinese herbal remedies are becoming increasingly popular and more widely available. We also recommend a visit to a practitioner of this system of medicine.

In traditional Chinese herbal medicine, diagnosis and treatment are based on a person's underlying constitutional type and deficiencies or imbalances in organ and energy systems. This vision of the whole patient forms the foundation on which the treatment plan is constructed. As the practitioner blends herbs to address the deficiencies and imbalances, there is also room to include Western herbal therapies.

Perhaps the example of the woman suffering from chronic bladder infections is most useful. Western herbalism suggests barberry, uva ursi leaf, and usnea lichen to clear the infection, plus demulcent herbs such as marshmallow root to soothe the mucous membrane that lines the bladder wall. While this treatment plan will clear the infection, it may not prevent recurrences.

Traditional Chinese Medicine focuses on addressing the underlying constitutional imbalance that creates the cycle of repeated infections. For example, the above case may be a result of "kidney Yin deficiency." Since the Yin aspect of the body is responsible for cooling and lubricating the organs, a deficiency of Yin can lead to overheating of a particular system. If the lack of Yin lubrication occurs in the kidneys, the urinary tract will be prone to chronic inflammation due to this overheating, in much the same way a car will overheat if it is low on oil and water.

The Yin cooling system of the kidneys can be depleted by stress, over-work, and environmental toxins. It can be replenished, however, by herbal formulas that nourish kidney Yin.

HOW TO TAKE HERBS

In most cases, the herbs suggested in this book can be taken as teas, tinctures, or pills; use whatever form is most convenient for you. With some herbs and formulas, one type of preparation may be more effective; we'll give you that information, but the best type of preparation for you is the one you are most likely to take consistently. This book offers formulas that you can blend yourself. You can also seek similar ones at your local health-food store. But the best formulas are custom designed for the individual. We hope this book will encourage you to blend your own.

One principle is true of herbs no matter what your constitution or ailment: Quality is important. Herbal preparations are only as good as the herbs themselves. Unless you have your own herb garden where you can be assured of good quality, purchase your herbs from a reputable store or mail-order business. Store dried herbs in airtight containers, preferably glass, away from heat and direct sunlight, which increase oxidation and cause dried herbs and essential oils to deteriorate. Keep leaves and flowers no more than a year; roots and barks remain potent for at least two or three years. The dried herbs you purchase should retain their taste, smell, and color, and fragrant plants should still have their characteristic aroma. For example, dried chamomile that is brown instead of yellow, or peppermint that has lost most of its smell, doesn't offer very strong medicine. You should return these herbs for a refund. Finely cut or powdered herbs lose their potency faster than ones that you purchase as whole leaves, flowers, bark, or berries. A guide to some of the types of herbal preparations recommended in this book follows.

Infusions and Decoctions

These preparations, often simply called teas, are the simplest and least expensive of all the ways to take herbs. Tea gives you a chance to befriend the

CULINARY CURES

Many traditional cuisines incorporate medicinal herbs, such as astragalus and codonopsis, into soups, stews, and other foods daily. Almost all the herbs and spices used to season foods have medicinal properties. For example, turmeric is an excellent liver protector and anti-inflammatory; cayenne clears the sinuses and boosts the metabolic rate; and aromatic herbs such as anise, caraway, and fennel are good for the digestion. Ginger is a sovereign remedy for nausea, whether it is due to PMS or pregnancy. Thyme and lavender have anti-bacterial properties, and garlic boosts the immune system and fights infections. Applications of these culinary remedies are discussed in the chapters on specific conditions.

herbs by smelling and tasting them, encouraging you to relax while you sip. Infusions and decoctions must be refrigerated, and even then they keep only a few days.

Infusions are made from tender leaves, stems, and flowers of medicinal plants. To make them, heat water just to boiling, then pour it over the herbs or immerse the herbs in the pot. Cover your cup, teapot or pan to keep the heat in, and steep the herbs for five to fifteen minutes. Then simply strain, reheat if necessary, and drink. Tea bags use more finely powdered herbs, so they do not need to be steeped as long. Use about 1 heaping teaspoon of herb for every cup of water, or a tea bag in a tea cup. A typical medicinal dose is one strong cup of tea, two to four times a day.

Decoctions are made from roots, barks, and berries; because these parts of a plant are tougher, the active compounds are more securely locked away, so more heat and time are required to release them. To make a decoction, gently simmer roots or barks in water fifteen to thirty minutes. Keep the heat extra low for aromatic roots such as valerian and angelica, so their essential oils aren't lost into the air.

Sometimes you will want to make a tea from a mixture of herbs that includes both types of plant parts. In that case, you can simmer the woody parts to make a decoction, then remove the pot from the heat and add the leaves and flowers. Cover and steep; then strain and drink.

Tinctures and Glycerites

Tinctures and glycerites, also called extracts, are concentrations of an herb's active chemicals in a base of alcohol (tinctures) or glycerin (glycerites). They offer several advantages over other ways to take herbs. The extract bottles are easy to carry and need no refrigeration. They keep for years and are easy for the body to assimilate. The concentrated form makes it easier to take large doses. Taking a tincture means that you ingest alcohol, although only a small amount: four average doses a day usually contain less than one teaspoon of alcohol. Glycerites avoid alcohol altogether, but they often are only half the potency of tinctures. Some active constituents do not extract into glycerin.

An average dose of a tincture or glycerite is about two to three droppersful, or about a quarter teaspoon. This amount roughly equals one cup of tea. A dose is generally taken three to six times a day. Some tinctures are prepared as "extra strength"; follow the manufacturer's recommendation when using these preparations.

Tablets and Capsules

Pills offer a fast and easy way to down even unpalatable herbs.

Although they act more slowly than tinctures, they are even more convenient to carry around. Since they are such a popular way to take herbs, you will find a large selection. It is more difficult to judge the freshness of pills, but when carefully stored in a cool place, they should last at least a year. Capsules contain powdered herbs enclosed in a gelatin or vegetable-based shell. Tablets are dried herbs, pressed and formed with binders such as cellulose. These products can vary considerably in strength, so read the labels carefully and follow the manufacturer's directions or your herbalist's instructions.

Standardized Extracts

Some modern research on herbs has focused on how they exert their healing effects. Sometimes a specific chemical component has been identified, such as the hypericin in St. John's wort. Because herbs are natural products, and their level of active constituents varies, supplement manufacturers have sought ways to assure customers that their products contain the beneficial compounds for which the herb is being taken. Standardized tinctures and pills are guaranteed to have a specific amount or percentage of an herb's active compound. Reputable manufacturers make sure that each batch of herbs they process contains enough of the primary active substance. If not, the pure active substances derived from that plant or another source are added to bring up the percentage in the product. But the percentage of active chemical is not necessarily the same from company to company. Always read the label carefully. Also, the way in which an herb acts on the body is always due to a synergy of many substances, not just one active one, so this process is controversial among herbalists. We feel that standardized products are useful sometimes, especially when most research on an herb's benefits for a specific condition also is based on a standardized extract.

A Word on Dosage

When you begin to take an herbal remedy, we advise starting with a small dose. While herbs work gently, they are still powerful substances; individuals may have sensitivities or allergies to them just as they do to other foods and drugs. If you find you have no sensitivities, slowly increase your dose, taking into account the severity of your condition and your body size. Most herbs have few, if any, side effects, so you do not need to take exactly thirty drops. However, some herbs, like some vitamins, can be harmful in large doses. If you believe you need to increase your dosage above what's recommended, you should consult a qualified practitioner.

ABOUT WOMEN'S HERBS

We use three main criteria to help us determine what herbs are likely to be most effective for preventing and healing women's diseases. The herb must have a long history that helps determine safe and effective use, dosage, and contraindications. We also look closely at the modern scientific work that has been performed. Finally, we must have some personal experience with the herb or know an experienced herbalist who does. Only then do we wholeheartedly recommend an herb or herbal formula to you.

The description of the women's herbs that follows is based on these guidelines. While some of these popular women's herbs have a long history of use, a few also are supported by recent human studies. They also are among the most widely used among present-day herbal practitioners.

We want to introduce you to a few herbs in detail—the ones that are especially important to women's health. It is a good idea to become familiar with them now, since you will encounter these same herbs over and over again in the following chapters. We've also included briefer information about additional women's herbs in the chart at the end of this chapter.

Black Cohosh *(Cimicifuga racemosa)*

Black cohosh was a common uterine tonic at the turn of the century, and was used to diminish false labor pains and regulate and increase true ones. It was also used to ease pain and help calm the nervous system after labor. For painful or delayed periods, Eclectic physician Dr. John King suggested combining black cohosh with cramp bark as early as 1876. Black cohosh is quickly regaining its popularity now that European doctors prescribe it to relieve hot flashes and for conditions caused by a lack of estrogen, such as depression during menopause. It must be taken over a period of time to be effective, and is often blended with vitex. Black cohosh is one of the most promising phytoestrogenic herbs, and is available in tinctures or standardized extracts in tablets and capsules. In Traditional Chinese Medicine, other species of black cohosh are used to treat prolapse of the uterus, fatigue, and shortness of breath.

Standard dose: Tincture, 10 to 60 drops, two or three times daily; decoction, one cup twice daily (decoctions usually combine black cohosh with other herbs); standardized extract, three capsules twice daily. Be sure to take three days off each month that you are taking the herb.

CAUTION: Although no contraindications have been found for black cohosh, we suggest not taking it for longer than four to six months. Avoid it during pregnancy except for two weeks before the due date, and even then it is best to seek professional guidance. Avoid high doses of this herb.

Cramp Bark *(Viburnum opulus)*

Cramp bark has long been used as a strong antispasmodic. It helps relieve cramping and irregular bleeding during the menstrual cycle and cramping that may occur during pregnancy and postpartum. It is used similarly to black haw as a miscarriage preventative. We find that blending cramp bark with equal parts of valerian can enhance its uterus-relaxing effects, relieving cramps more effectively.

The related herb, black haw *(Viburnum prunifolium)* is also a favorite herb to prevent miscarriage. The herb is also used for painful menstruation in deficiency conditions, where bleeding is scanty, and debility and nervousness are present, and for lower back and "bearing down" pains. Other indications for black haw include leg cramps due to pregnancy or other causes. It is sometimes used for excessive uterine bleeding during menopause.

Standard dose: Tincture, three to five droppersful, three to five times daily; infusion, two or three cups daily as needed.

Dong Quai *(Angelica sinensis)*

Dong quai root is said to be one of the most widely used herbs in the world. It is well-known for its ability to tonify the blood and uterus. It helps relieve insufficient, painful, and irregular menstruation and symptoms of PMS, menopause, and uterine fibroids. In some cases, it also promotes fertility, especially when infertility is caused by lack of uterine tone. During menopause, formulas containing dong quai can be used to help alleviate symptoms such as fatigue and vaginal dryness. It can increase menstrual and intermittent bleeding in some women. Furthermore, be aware that Chinese practitioners almost never give dong quai by itself, but combine it with other herbs to help balance its warm and spicy aspects. Even in formulas for menopause, dong quai is often one of seven or eight other herbs.

Standard dose: Tincture, one to two droppersful twice daily; decoction, one cup two or three times daily. Take for up to nine months; if desired, take a three-day break each month.

CAUTION: Do not take dong quai during pregnancy.

Motherwort *(Leonurus cardiaca)*

Motherwort has long been used for suppressed, irregular, or painful menstruation and to calm the nervous system. Motherwort increases blood flow to tissues, especially the heart muscle; herbalists believe that it helps regulate the heart's actions. It also helps regulate menstrual flow. In certain cases and in combination with other herbs, such as vitex and false unicorn root, it may support fertility. It also may help shrink fibroids but can increase menstrual flow; women with heavy bleeding may want to avoid it, or substitute a different herb in formulas that contain it.

Standard dose: Tincture, one to two droppersful two or three times daily; decoction, one cup two or three times daily. Take for the same duration as dong quai.

CAUTION: Avoid motherwort during pregnancy.

Red Raspberry *(Rubus idaeus)*

Probably the best known use for raspberry leaf is to tone the uterus during pregnancy and to facilitate labor. We have heard hundreds of women attest to its efficacy when taken for several months. A red raspberry tea can be frozen in ice cube trays and given to women in labor to suck on to strengthen their contractions. It is also said to reduce pain and uterine swelling and to minimize bleeding after childbirth. However, raspberry is useful for far more than childbirth. Its toning action on the uterus makes it an important remedy for most uterine conditions and to improve the health and strength of the uterus before pregnancy. We include it in formulas for miscarriage prevention, combined with wild yam, false unicorn root, and other herbs. Some European doctors recommend drinking red raspberry leaf tea to alleviate morning sickness. It can also help relieve pain and excessive bleeding during menstruation and help to correct uterine prolapse.

Standard dose: One or two cups of the tea, two or three times daily. Take for the same duration as dong quai.

Vitex *(Vitex agnus-castus)*

Vitex has become one of the most widely known of all women's herbs and is certainly one of our all-time favorites. It was recommended by Hippocrates in 450 B.C., and remains the most popular European herbal remedy for PMS and menopausal symptoms. Scientists think that vitex works by regulating the pituitary gland, which sends chemical signals to other glands telling them how much of each particular hormone to make. Vitex is used for easing symptoms of PMS, menopause, fibroid cysts, irregular menstrual cycles, and to increase fertility. In Europe, women use vitex to help normalize menstruation and ovulation when they discontinue taking birth control pills. When used regularly, vitex may help moderate mood swings, relieve depression, and ease food cravings. Clinical research shows that vitex may begin working after only ten days, but to see its full benefits, it should be taken for at least six months. It is also used to increase the supply of milk in nursing mothers. It is often combined with black cohosh.

Standard dose: Tincture, one or two droppersful first thing in the morning or morning and evening for stubborn conditions; capsules, two to five grams daily. Take for about six months.

CAUTION: Do not take vitex during pregnancy except under the guidance of an experienced herbalist. This herb may lessen the effectiveness of birth control pills.

Yarrow *(Achillea millefolium)*

Yarrow has been used to treat menstrual pain, heavy periods, postpartum bleeding, and both incontinence and suppression of urine. It is also used to tonify the urinary system, particularly when the uterus is weak or excessive bleeding occurs near the onset of menopause, after childbirth, or after miscarriage. The German Commission E lists yarrow to treat cramps.

Standard dose: Tincture, twenty to forty drops two or three times daily; infusion, one cup two or three times daily. Use as needed.

CAUTION: Yarrow is contraindicated for persons allergic to plants in the Compositae (formerly Asteraceae) family.

ADDITIONAL WOMEN'S HERBS

Herb	Conditions	Chapter
Alfalfa (*Medicago sativa*)	Anemia, osteoporosis, high cholesterol	3, 15, 16
Artichoke (*Cynara scolymus*)	High cholesterol, liver and bile stagnation, poor digestion	2, 6, 8, 12, 15
Barberry (*Berberis vulgaris*)	Urinary tract infections, trichamoniasis	9, 10, 11
Bilberry (*Vaccinum myrtillus*)	Fragile capillaries, varicose veins	10
Black haw (*Viburnum prunifolium*)	Menstrual pain, inflammation	5
Black walnut (*Juglans nigra*)	Yeast infections	9
Boldo (*Peumus boldo*)	Cystitis, liver congestion, mood swings due to liver congestion	5, 6, 7

Herb	Conditions	Chapter
Burdock (*Arctium lappa*)	PMS, fibroids, anemia	2, 3, 4, 6, 7, 8, 9, 12
Butcher's broom (*Ruscus aculeatus*)	Varicose veins	15
Cactus (*Selinicereus grandiflorus*)	Heart problems such as palpitations, irregular heartbeat	15
Calendula (*Calendula officinalis*)	Cervical dysplasia, breast cysts, menstrual pain	5, 7, 8, 9
Chamomile, German (*Matricaria recutita*)	Cramps, breast cysts, PMS, nervousness,	4, 5, 6, 7, 8, 9, 14, 15
Chaparral (*Larrea divaricata*)	Trichamoniasis, dysplasia	7, 12
Cleavers (*Galium aparine*)	Uterine fibroids, breast cysts, lymphatic congestion	7, 8
Coptis (*Coptis chinensis*)	Yeast infections, trichamoniasis	9
Corn silk (*Zea mays*)	Bladder and urinary tract infections	10
Cranberry (*Vaccinum macrocarpon*)	Urinary tract infections	10
Dandelion (*Taraxacum officinale*)	PMS, anemia, liver congestion	3, 5, 6, 8, 9, 12
Echinacea (*Echinacea purpurea, E. angustifolia*)	Yeast and other types of infections	9, 11
Evening primrose (*Oenethera biennis*)	PMS, breast tenderness, menstrual cramps	5, 6, 8, 14
False unicorn root (*Chamaelirium luteum*)	Heavy periods, inflammation, cramps	5, 7
Flax seeds (meal and oil) (*Linum usitissamum*)	Bladder irritation, constipation, PMS, vaginal dryness, vaginal atrophy after menopause	5, 10, 14
Garlic (*Allium sativum*)	Vaginal infections, high blood pressure, high cholesterol	5, 9, 10, 15
Ginger (*Zingiber officinalis*)	Suppressed menstruation, pelvic congestion, menstrual pain, nausea	5, 6, 12, 13
Ginkgo (*Ginkgo biloba*)	Poor circulation, headache and breast tenderness associated with PMS, poor memory, depression	4, 6, 15
Ginseng (*Panax ginseng*)	Menopause, poor digestion, low energy	4, 14

Herb	Conditions	Chapter
Goldenrod (*Solidago virgaurea*)	Cystitis, irritated bladder, missed periods	10, 15
Goldenseal (*Hydrastis canadensis*)	Bladder infections, uterine bleeding, trichamoniasis, yeast infections	9
Green tea (*Camellia sinensis*)	High cholesterol, heart disease and cancer prevention	7, 15
Hawthorn (*Crataegus laevigata*)	Palpitations, angina, hypertension, irregular heartbeat	15
Horse chestnut (*Aesculus hippocastunum*)	Varicose veins, bruises, hemorrhoids, venous insufficiency	15
Horsetail (*Equisetum arvense*)	Bladder infections, excessive menstrual bleeding, weak or brittle bones, nails, hair	7, 8, 10, 15, 16
Juniper (*Juniperus communis*)	Bladder infections	6, 10, 12
Lavender (*Lavandula officinalis*)	Vaginal infections, depression, anxiety	4, 5, 6, 7, 8, 9, 11, 13, 14
Lemon balm (*Melissa officinalis*)	Anxiety, tension, herpes	4, 11, 14, 15
Licorice (*Glycyrrhiza glabra*)	Bladder infections, adrenal depletion, viral infections, chronic fatigue	3, 4, 5, 6, 11, 14
Linden (*Tilia europa*)	High cholesterol, hypertension	4, 14, 15
Marshmallow (*Althea officinalis*)	Bladder and urinary tract irritation	9, 10
Milk thistle (*Silybum marianum*)	Liver stress or damage	2, 4, 5, 8, 9, 11, 12
Mugwort (*Artemisia vulgaris*)	Missed periods, menstrual pain, bile stagnation	8, 15
Mullein (*Verbascum thapsis*)	Uterine fibroids, breast cysts, lymphatic congestion, lung problems	7, 8
Myrrh (*Commiphora molmol*)	Bladder infections	7, 10, 11, 15
Nettles (*Urtica dioica*)	Anemia, excessive bleeding	3, 5, 15, 16
Oregon grape (*Berberis aquifolium*)	Yeast infections, urinary tract infections, acne	9, 10, 12
Osha (*Ligusticum porteri*)	Missed periods, colds	9, 10
Parsley root (*Petroselinum crispum*)	Missed periods, urinary tract infections	6, 10
Partridge berry (*Mitchella repens*)	Menstrual pain, irregular periods, prolapsed uterus	5

Herb	Conditions	Chapter
Pau d'arco (*Tabebuia* spp.)	Yeast infections	9
Pipsissewa (*Chimaphila umbellata*)	Bladder and urinary tract infections	10
Plantain (*Plantago lanceolata*)	Bladder infections, skin inflammation, bites, stings, burns	7, 8, 10, 11, 13
Prickly ash bark (*Xanthoxylum americanum*)	Uterine fibroids	5, 8
Red clover (*Trifolium pratense*)	Cervical dysplasia, osteoporosis, menopause	5, 7, 12, 14, 16
Reishi (*Ganoderma lucidum*)	Heart problems, high cholesterol, insomnia, nervousness, agitation	4, 9, 10, 12, 14, 15
Rosemary (*Rosmarinus officinalis*)	Vaginal infections, missed periods	5, 7, 9, 12
Sarsaparilla (*Smilax* spp.)	Syphilis, skin problems	12
Saw palmetto (*Serenoa serrulata*)	Urinary, uterine, and vaginal conditions; frequent urination	7, 10, 14
Slippery elm (*Ulmus rubra*)	Bladder infections, vaginal infections	9
St. John's wort (*Hypericum perforatum*)	Mood swings associated with PMS and menopause; vaginal dryness (oil form)	4, 6, 11, 14
Tea tree (*Malaleuca alternifolia*)	Vaginal yeast and other infections	9, 10, 11, 12
Thyme (*Thymus vulgaris*)	Vaginal yeast and other infections	5, 9
Turmeric (*Curcuma longa*)	Liver stress	4, 5, 9, 12
Usnea (*Usnea* spp.)	Urinary tract infections, trichamoniasis	10
Witch hazel (*Hamamelis* spp.)	Hemorrhoids, varicose veins	15
Wormwood (*Artemisia absinthium*)	Liver stagnation, trichamoniasis	6, 9
Yellow dock (*Rumex crispus*)	Anemia, pregnancy	3, 4, 5, 7

Chapter 2

WOMEN'S HORMONES

*Hormones take a lot of the heat for women's health complaints.
But nearly every woman, armed with information about how
hormones work, can use natural healing methods to exert some
control over her own hormonal balance.*

Hormones are chemical messengers that have a specific regulatory effect on the activity of organs, cells and tissues. They are produced in the endocrine glands, such as the ovaries, and travel through the blood to their target tissue. Meanwhile, the endocrine system, the body's collection of glands, works with the nervous system to regulate homeostasis, or the healthy balance of the body. It's these chemical messengers that cause the development of sexual characteristics, regulate menstruation, or prepare a women's body to carry a child. Hormones probably affect emotions, too. Science is just beginning to understand how these complex reactions inside the body influence immunity, reproductive behavior, disease, and health. But most women can exert some healing influence over their own hormonal balance. In order to do so, it's first important to understand what the major women's hormones do and how they are affected by various drug and natural therapies.

There are three general classes of hormones:

Steroid hormones include the sex hormones, which are fat-soluble molecules that the body fashions from cholesterol. These hormones include estrogen, progesterone, and testosterone; they are produced in the ovaries and, during pregnancy, the placenta.

Amino-acid-derived hormones are water-soluble molecules, smaller than steroid hormones. They include the "fight or flight" hormones epinephrine and norepinephrine, released by the adrenal glands when a human or other animal encounters a threatening situation, and thyroid hormones such as thyroxin.

Protein-based hormones are a complex and diverse group of chemicals. Examples include insulin from the pancreas and the hormones from the anterior lobe of the pituitary gland, such as growth hormone, thyroid-stimulating hormone, and gonadotropic hormone. Each of these hormones has unique structural characteristics that make it possible for each of them to exert a specific physiological effect.

THE MAJOR WOMEN'S HORMONES

Hormones are continuously secreted, usually in small amounts. There are more than fifty different hormones. Hormone secretion is highly regulated so that each hormone is produced only when it is needed. Hormones connect with their target tissues like a lock and key; only a specific hormone may attach to the tissue at specific receptor cells. Some tissues have receptor cells for more than one hormone; for instance, cells in the uterine lining can receive both estrogen and progesterone.

A woman's physical and emotional well-being, her physical endurance, her reproductive capacity, and her sex drive rely on a delicate balance of hormones. Hormone levels fluctuate throughout the month and even during the day. Blood tests for hormone levels detect only the blood-borne hormones, not those held in the body's tissues. Some women ride their natural hormonal changes like the crest of a wave, but others may feel more like they are being pulled into the undertow.

Estrogen

Estrogen, the primary female hormone, is produced in three different types: estradiol, estriol, and estrone. In concert with other hormones such as progesterone and growth hormone, estrogen stimulates the development of secondary female sex characteristics such as breasts and labia. From approximately the fourth day after menstruation, estrogen levels increase to a peak just before ovulation around the thirteenth day. This estrogenic peak signals the uterine lining, or endometrium, to thicken in anticipation of pregnancy. Then, after ovulation, estrogen levels plummet. During the menstrual cycle's second half, progesterone is the dominant hormone, with estrogen increasing again but remaining secondary. Progesterone further prepares the endometrium to accept a fertilized egg cell. If that fertilization and implantation does not occur, estrogen and progesterone levels drop and the endometrium breaks down and is shed during a new menstrual cycle.

Estrogen exerts many beneficial physical changes in women. The hormone stimulates the oil glands of the skin and scalp, making skin and hair softer and silkier. It also improves the tone of blood vessels and improves circulation to the uterus. Yet overabundant estrogen is associated with conditions such as endometriosis, uterine fibroids, breast cysts, and endometrial and breast cancers. PMS and irregular menstruation may also be related.

Prolactin

The main job of prolactin is to prepare the body, especially the breasts, for nursing a child. But several studies have implicated an abnormal production of this hormone in menstrual irregularities, such as water retention and breast soreness.

THE NEWS ABOUT DHEA

Dehydroepiandrosterone, or DHEA, is an adrenal hormone that is abundant in the young. Those age 80, however, have only a tenth of the hormone that they had at age 25. This has led many to assume that DHEA is linked with the disorders of aging such as wrinkled skin, arthritis, memory loss, heart disease, and even cancer. Some have suggested that supplements of DHEA will prevent or cure these problems and even extend lifespan by 50 percent. In the body, DHEA is a weak hormone that is less active than testosterone. In premenopausal women, DHEA competes with estrogen and limits its actions, but in postmenopausal women DHEA is more likely to act as estrogen. In other words, it performs a balancing act in the body. Its ability to change roles is probably why some studies show that it protects against some forms of cancer while others find it promotes them.

In a study sponsored by the National Cancer Institute, high blood levels of DHEA in postmenopausal women were found to correlate with significantly elevated risk of developing breast cancer when compared to otherwise similar women. A recent British study found that despite many claims that DHEA prevents cardiovascular disease, in fact it yields no benefit. In addition, high doses may cause side effects such as acne, unwanted hair growth, irritability, insomnia, low energy, and a deepened voice. So much remains unknown about DHEA that we feel that people should not use it without the advice and supervision of a health-care practitioner. Women with normal levels should avoid it.

Progesterone

Progesterone's primary job is to prepare the uterus for fertilization and prevent the uterine contractions that might expel a fetus. It is produced mostly by the corpus luteum, the mature follicle from which an egg cell is released each month; very minute amounts are also produced by the adrenal glands. Progesterone levels begin to increase after ovulation, peaking midway through the second half of the cycle.

If a woman does become pregnant, the placenta that develops around the fetus produces high levels of progesterone as well as estrogen throughout the pregnancy, as much as fifteen times the normal level. Progesterone acts with prolactin and estrogen to stimulate breast development and produce milk. It also increases the availability of oxygen to the uterus.

In nonpregnant women, excess progesterone reduces and thickens vaginal secretions and causes vaginal dryness, swelling, and itching. It may also result in a longer, but scantier menstrual period and spotting between periods. Excess progesterone slows the body down and contributes to fatigue, muscle aches, reduced libido, weight gain, and increased appetite. Low progesterone levels, on the other hand, may result in frequent, heavy periods or none at all and may contribute to PMS.

Testosterone

Testosterone is usually referred to as the "male" hormone, but women's bodies also produce it in small quantities. In women, it's manufactured by the ovaries, the liver, and the adrenal glands. The brain's testosterone receptors are located in areas involved with sex and emotion; the hormone seems to be associated with energy, sex drive, love, and lust. Testosterone peaks twice a month, once just before menstruation and again before ovulation. It is especially high in women taking birth control pills. Testosterone rises in women (but not in men) after they drink a couple of glasses of wine.

In many postmenopausal women, total testosterone levels do not drop very much; the ovaries and other glands continue to manufacture it. When symptoms such as low sex drive occur and a blood-hormone test for testosterone shows low levels, testosterone replacement is sometimes recommended.

Testosterone supplements come in a variety of forms, including pills, liquid solution, a gel to rub on the skin, and pellets that are implanted under the skin. Testosterone's side effects may include liver disease, increased facial hair, and occasionally acne, a deepening of the voice, and enlargement of the clitoris.

HORMONE HELPERS

Herbal therapies can help you move gracefully through hormonal changes. While herbs do not supply the same hormones as the human body, some do have phytohormones—compounds that can influence human hormones or the tissues that hormones normally target. These phytohormones work differently than supplementation with human hormones. They may mimic, activate, or block a hormone's action, or help to make the target tissues less sensitive to hormones.

Herbs that contain phytoestrogen and other hormone regulators often take time to relieve symptoms and restore balance. Their effects on the body are neither as immediate nor as abrupt as most pharmaceutical drugs; they assist natural processes in a gradual but powerful way. Herbs also contain vitamins, minerals, and antioxidants that the body can use to heal itself. This is not to say that all herbs, just because they are natural, are safe when taken in any amount. For example, foxglove contains compounds that can fatally overstimulate the heart, and belladonna contains an alkaloid called atropine that can powerfully affect the nervous system. But after thirty years of observing how herbs work, we have seen very few adverse reactions. We feel confident about the safety and effectiveness of herbs, especially when they are used with knowledge.

The Liver and Hormones

What does the health of your liver have to do with hormones and hormone-related complaints? Plenty. The liver is the organ that makes sure the body is able to absorb the nutrients it needs and get rid of waste products, toxins, and excess hormones. It acts as a filter for the blood, stores some vitamins and minerals, and creates enzymes, cholesterol, and bile, which help break down foods and fats. Bile salts also contain cholesterol, the raw material for steroid hormones. According to Traditional Chinese Medicine, the liver regulates the blood and harmonizes the emotions. But it's the liver's relationship to estrogen that is the key to its role in women's health. The liver breaks down excess estrogen so that it can be excreted by the digestive tract. Overabundant hormones can actually damage the liver as it tries to cope with the overload. Excess hormones are often to blame in many women's symptoms and disorders, including PMS, endometriosis, breast cysts, uterine fibroids, and possibly some types of cancer.

There are several ways you can keep your liver healthy. One of the best strategies is to keep alcohol consumption to a minimum. If you do overindulge once in a while, red ginseng, evening primrose oil, and borage

MAKING SENSE OF PROGESTERONE PRODUCTS

During the last few years, creams made with progesterone have been promoted as curing everything from vaginal dryness to alcoholism. Promoters of these creams even say that the hormone reduces stress by making a woman feel more emotionally content. Science, however, shows only that oral progesterone supplementation may help a woman build bone, and that a deficiency may be a factor in bone loss after menopause. Some evidence indicates that it may be easier for some women to conceive with vaginal cream application. Progesterone creams or supplements also may reduce unpleasant symptoms of PMS, such as water retention (see the PMS chapter for more information). Meanwhile, consumers can choose from a variety of over-the-counter products that make progesterone-like claims. Many of these creams contain wild yam extract derived from the species *Dioscora villosa, D. paniculata, D. mexicana,* or others. This extract contains diosgenin, from which drug companies synthesize a variety of hormones, including estrogens, progesterone, progestin, and testosterone.

Diosgenin itself, however, has not been proven to have any hormonal activity in the human body, although promoters of these creams quote testimonials of wondrous results. In addition, the creams contain widely varying amounts of progesterone, from 25 mg per ounce to 400 mg per ounce. Newer products contain micronized progesterone, very fine suspended droplets of hormone; high doses are required to prevent the liver from breaking it down. Recently micronized progesterone creams containing 100 mg per ounce have been shown effective in protecting the uterus without interfering with estrogen; in addition, it increases "good" cholesterol, HDL, while decreasing the "bad" cholesterol, LDL. It may also fight osteoporosis by helping to build bone (instead of stopping resorption like estrogen does). Used alone, it may relieve hot flashes. Progesterone is metabolized and deactivated at different rates in each individual, so its effectiveness may vary.

Although it is more expensive than creams containing progestins, the micronized progesterone creams' only side effect is drowsiness. Progestin creams, on the other hand, can cause depression, fatigue, bloating, and breast tenderness. So what's a consumer to do? It's best to use these creams only under the advice of your health-care practitioner because the products vary so widely. If you do decide to try them, read the labels and buy carefully in small amounts. Claims that seem too good to be true probably are.

seed oil may help purify your blood and ease the burden on your liver. Milk thistle can help repair the damage that's already been done.

Nutritional supplements play a role in liver health. Vitamins E and C can increase its health and efficiency. Choline, inositol, and the amino acid methionine also help the liver convert and emulsify not only fat itself, but fat-soluble hormones like estrogen. Look for nutritional supplements that contain these compounds.

Finally, liver herbs may help even hard-to-treat women's health problems like PMS. These herbs can neutralize substances that harm the liver, reduce or help repair damage that has already occurred, increase production of beneficial liver enzymes, and generally make the liver operate more efficiently.

Here is a sampling of important liver herbs that subsequent chapters will mention in detail.

- Liver protectors and rebuilders include milk thistle, schisandra, ginger, turmeric, and artichoke-leaf and grape seed extract.

- Liver cleansers include dandelion root, lemon juice, yellow dock root, burdock root, and boldo. The following recipe will help you purify and strengthen your liver and will boost any other therapy that you undertake.

Liver-Boosting Tea

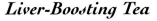

3 teaspoons burdock root
1 teaspoon dandelion root
1/2 teaspoon schisandra berries
1/2 teaspoon licorice root
1/2 teaspoon ginger root
1 quart water

Add herbs to water; heat to a simmer for 2 minutes. Turn down the heat and allow to steep for 15 minutes. Strain out herbs. Drink at least two cups a day. This tea, like the others in this book, can be made ahead and refrigerated for up to three days.

CHAPTER 3

ANEMIA

Even when a lack of iron causes no serious health problems, it can prevent a woman from enjoying her full potential.

Anemia is not a disease, but rather a condition that can result in a group of symptoms: pallor, fatigue, vertigo, headache, ringing in the ears, a racing or irregular heartbeat, an inability to catch one's breath after physical exertion. Anemic women are typically pale and often tired, weak, or dizzy; they fall asleep easily. They may be prone to headaches and digestive disturbances. In extreme cases, anemia sufferers can experience chest pain or even heart failure. What's happening? The body is failing to deliver enough oxygen to its cells, either because of a shortage of red cells or a reduction of hemoglobin. For sufferers, this can mean lost vitality, lowered resistance to disease, poor performance on mental tasks, and in general a lower quality of health.

Anemia's causes fall into four basic categories: deficient nutrients in the diet, or deficient absorption of them; bleeding or blood loss (from menstruation, a bleeding ulcer, or other causes); decreased red blood cell production; or increased red blood destruction. In some of these cases, the hemoglobin molecules—the carrier molecules within the red blood cells that actually transport oxygen—are impaired in some way.

Several hereditary defects can impair the hemoglobin molecule, resulting in sickle-cell anemia or another inherited anemia called thalassemia. Systemic diseases or infections that may be undetected—such as asymptomatic colon cancer or rheumatoid arthritis—can also lead to anemia. For this reason, when interviews and initial blood tests fail to trace the cause of a patient's anemia, doctors often order further tests, perhaps even a biopsy of the bone marrow where blood cells are produced.

The most common anemia women have is iron deficiency. Deficiencies of other nutrients can cause anemia as well. Vitamin B12 deficiency anemia, also called pernicious anemia, can occur with poor diet, some vegetarian diets, or poor

Yellow dock

absorption of this vitamin. Anemia resulting from folic acid deficiency is even more common, and can be caused by poor diet or absorption, pregnancy, or alcoholism.

IRON DEFICIENCY AND ANEMIA

Doctors define iron deficiency as a serum ferritin level (the amount of iron stored in the blood) of less than 12 micrograms per liter. If iron levels remain low for weeks or months, the condition can progress into iron-deficient anemia. At this point, there is insufficient iron in the body for the bone marrow to build new red blood cells.

A 1997 study found that between 9 and 11 percent of American women of childbearing age were iron deficient. Between 2 and 5 percent were anemic.

Iron deficiency is most likely to happen at certain times of life—infancy, adolescence, pregnancy, and nursing. It can also happen simply because of heavy menstrual periods. A study published by the National Center for Health Statistics, a branch of the Centers for Disease Control and Prevention, found that between 9 and 11 percent of American women of childbearing age were iron deficient. Between 2 and 5 percent had iron-deficiency anemia. A regional office of the World Health Organization calls iron deficiency anemia one of the major micronutrient deficiencies worldwide.

Even when iron deficiency isn't causing overt symptoms, it can prevent a woman from enjoying her full potential. A study of apparently healthy teenagers shows that low hemoglobin levels have an adverse effect on physical performance. Anemia may even affect memory. A 1991 study at the University of Texas Medical Branch in Galveston shows that women who take iron supplements score up to 20 percent higher on memory tests than those who take no iron.

Considerations for Pregnant Women

Because of greater demands on a woman's body during pregnancy, childbirth, and the early months of caring for a child, pregnant and nursing women are at special risk for deficiency anemias. Folic acid deficiency is a common—and worrisome—phenomenon during pregnancy, because it has been linked with infant birth defects such as spina bifida, a type of neural tube defect in which the vertebrae don't completely close around the spinal cord. Over 70 percent of neural tube defects can be avoided by adequate amounts of folic acid taken during pregnancy.

To avoid these risks, supplements of iron, folic acid, and vitamin B12 are routinely recommended for pregnant women and those planning to become pregnant.

Some researchers, however, disagree with routine iron supplementation for pregnant women. In one study, the children born to a group of 1,330 healthy pregnant women who took extra iron were more than twice as likely to be hospitalized for convulsions than the children of 1,352 women who took iron only when their hemoglobin fell to a certain level. The researchers speculate that exposing the brain of the fetus to increased amounts of iron can make it more susceptible to injury or infection.

Research continues on how much iron is enough. A controlled study of 90 pregnant women conducted at the University of Bergen, Norway evaluated blood-iron levels in women who received only 27 mg of elemental iron. After pregnancy, the number of women in the placebo group whose iron stores were depleted was more than doubled; in the group of women receiving the iron supplement, the number with depleted iron stores was nearly halved.

WHAT A DOCTOR WILL DO

Testing for Anemia

Because anemia's symptoms can be an indication of other severe conditions, those who have them should consult their health care professional before beginning a self-treatment program. The most common test a doctor will order for checking the overall status of your blood is the complete blood count (CBC). The CBC measures the number of red and white blood cells, the level of hemoglobin in the blood, and other factors. One key measure included in the CBC is the hematocrit, which is a measure of the packed cell volume of red cells, expressed as a percentage of the total blood volume. The hematocrit is a measure that remains stable whether the red blood cells themselves are enlarged or shrunken, as can happen in some kinds of anemia. Be aware that the blood measures in the CBC can be affected by many things: smoking, altitude, and illnesses, to name a few.

Depending on other factors, a doctor may also order one of the following tests: serum ferritin, serum iron, total iron binding capacity, serum vitamin B12, folic acid, reticulocyte count, or a red blood cell fragility test. The serum ferritin test is a measure of how much iron is stored in the blood. Because anemia can signal an undiagnosed disease, doctors may even order a bone-marrow biopsy.

The metamorphosis of cells in the bone marrow into red blood cells, hemoglobin-packed and flattened to fit through tiny capillaries.

Medical Treatment

For iron deficient or anemic women, the most common conventional treatment is iron supplements. For healthy pregnant women, iron, B12, and folic acid supplements are often prescribed as a matter of routine. But questions about the effectiveness of supplements, the body's ability to absorb them, and the side effects of high iron levels in the blood have led some researchers to a cautious position.

The body's mechanism for absorbing iron is complex. In a 1994 study, some medical professionals recommended as much as 60 to 120 mg of iron per day, along with a multivitamin containing zinc and copper. But they found that iron was more effective if taken in a dose separate from the zinc and copper. The same study found that other supplements, such as calcium and magnesium, interfered with iron absorption. When the calcium carbonate in a multivitamin supplement was reduced from 350 to 250 mg, or the magnesium oxide reduced from 100 mg to 25 mg, iron absorption doubled. Another study found that iron absorption dropped 30 to 50 percent when the supplement was given with calcium.

On the other hand, supplementation can be orchestrated to help iron uptake rather than hinder it. Two studies have demonstrated that a combination of folic acid, vitamin B12, and iron is much more effective than iron alone. Researchers are divided on whether vitamin C helps iron absorption.

High Iron Levels and Health Risks

Above-normal iron levels have been found to have negative side effects sufficient to cause concern. The most minor include constipation, stomach distress, and depletion of vitamin E stores in the body. One theory holds that high amounts of iron in the blood can increase the chance of a woman developing heart disease, because the iron increases oxidation of LDL, the "bad" cholesterol, and thus initiates clogged arteries. Several studies have linked high blood-iron levels to an increased risk of infection. Some pathogens feed on iron in the blood; higher-than-necessary iron levels may simply give these bacteria and fungi more food.

The conclusion? Iron supplements are not a cure-all for iron deficiency or iron-deficiency anemia. To be sure that supplements are effective, women need to pay close attention to how they take them, when they take them, and with what food and other supplements. Over-supplementation carries its own risks and problems.

NATURAL HEALING

Anemia and Traditional Chinese Medicine

What is known as anemia in Western medicine is a more encompassing concept in Traditional Chinese Medicine. In this view of the body and its systems, blood is considered the "river of life" because it carries life-giving substances to every cell of the body: immune cells, hormones, nutrients, carrier proteins that transport hormones and other regulatory substances, and of course, oxygen. This river also carries away waste products such as carbon dioxide from all of the tissues, cells, and organs.

In Traditional Chinese Medicine, when the blood is weak and cannot perform its jobs, the condition is called "blood deficiency." It refers to more than simple anemia, and though it is more common in women than in men, both can develop it.

Maintaining a strong digestion, a healthy diet, and a strong liver are all part of a process that creates strong, vital blood and keeps it moving properly. Healthy blood is built from the nutrients in food, processed by the digestive tract. That food builds strong muscles and vital energy. When the digestion is weak—or if a large portion of the diet consists of empty, highly processed food—then the blood will also be weak.

In this view of the body, blood consists of more than iron and red blood cells. The liver stores blood and makes sure blood flows smoothly throughout the body. The symptoms of blood deficiency, however, mirror those observed in a medical context: fatigue, pale skin, mental weakness, poor memory, and dizziness. Other symptoms that Chinese medicine practitioners look for include dry eyes (the blood is said to moisten the eyes) and a pale tongue.

Dietary Changes

Just how important is diet in building strong blood with good oxygen-carrying capacity? Most practitioners of natural medicine agree that it is one of the single most important factors. They routinely emphasize diet and dietary supplements for women who may be iron deficient or who have anemia.

The best food sources of iron include sea vegetables (dulse, kelp, nori, etc.), beans, red meat, dried fruit, chicken, and seeds. Whole grains, green leafy vegetables (kale, beet greens, chard), and fish contain slightly less iron but are good sources when eaten regularly.

FOODS THAT INCREASE IRON ABSORPTION

Vitamin C

Fermented soybean products such as miso

Poultry

Fish

Red meat

Yogurt

Sauerkraut

In Traditional Chinese Medicine, meat is considered both a medicine and a food. For women who are feeling weak, fatigued, and generally deficient, it may be advisable to add a little chicken, fish, or red meat to the diet two to three times per week for moderate deficiency and daily for severe deficiency. They should continue eating it for several months to a year, depending on the severity of the deficiency. Vegetarians also can boost their dietary iron intake; it simply takes more meticulous diet planning.

Just as some vitamins and minerals can block the absorption of iron from iron supplements, some foods can diminish the effectiveness of iron-rich meals. Avoid consuming coffee, tea, zinc or manganese supplements, soy-protein powders (moderate amounts of whole soy products such as tofu are okay), bran, eggs, milk, calcium-rich antacids, or calcium supplements along with your iron-rich meal.

FOODS THAT INHIBIT IRON ABSORPTION
Bran in cereal and breads
Tea, coffee, and other caffeinated drinks
Calcium-rich antacids
Eggs
Milk and milk products
Some whole grains, especially when uncooked
Soy protein, especially soy milk, tofu, and soy protein

Diet issues for vegetarians

Are vegetarians more prone to anemia than people who eat red meat regularly? Based on our experience and a number of clinical studies, this association is not as certain as one might think. The overall quality and variety of the diet may be more important than whether one chooses to eat meat. However, it is probably easier to build strong blood with the aid of a little red meat, especially in people who are highly deficient. The iron that is found in meat, poultry, and fish is more easily absorbed by the body than the form of iron found in vegetarian sources.

WILD GREENS: NATURE'S VITAMIN PILLS

(milligrams of nutrient per 1/2 cup chopped raw greens)

Wild Green	Iron	Magnesium	Potassium	Zinc	Calcium	Phosphorus	Copper
Dandelion	0.87	10	111	0.20	52	18	0.11
Lamb's quarters	0.63	—	522	0.79	172	41	—
Nettles	1.20	28	132	0.34	117	23	.05
Yellow dock	1.61	69	261	—	42	25	—

Source: Pennington, 1994; Duke, 1992.

Many vegetarians turn to soy products, milk, and cheese to provide both protein and calcium in their diet—to the detriment of their iron intake. Soy products tend to inhibit iron absorption, especially soy protein powder. A 1994 study found that when vegetarian women—or women who simply avoid red meat—consume milk products daily, they are more likely to be both iron-deficient and zinc-deficient. For the most part, blood-building recommendations for vegetarians are the same as for omnivores—but they must be aware that some common meat substitutes block iron absorption and remember to eat them separately from high-iron meals.

Dietary iron boosters

In both Eastern and Western herbalism, wild greens and other chlorophyll-rich foods are thought of as boosters for healthy blood—though it's not exactly known how they work. In any case, the plants contain a rich supply of important minerals, including iron, magnesium, potassium, calcium, and zinc. Nettle greens also contain about 3.5 percent high-quality, complete protein.

The most potent way to use fresh nettle greens is to gather them in your area in the spring. A second growth in the late summer and early fall often appears, especially if greens are harvested in the spring. Remember to wear gloves to protect your hands, and cut only the top succulent stems with four to five pairs of leaves. If nettles are not growing in your area when you need them, buy some nettle tea at your local health food store. Other wild greens that boost the blood include dock greens, dandelion, and lamb's quarters. Squeezing some fresh lemon juice or adding a tablespoon of tasty vinegar to a dish of greens increases iron absorption—and tastes great, too. Lactic acid, found in yogurt, sauerkraut, and other fermented foods also boosts iron uptake.

SUPPLEMENT RECOMMENDATIONS

One respected text, M. R. Werbach's *Nutritional Influences on Illness*, suggests supplements in the following ranges for women suffering from iron deficiency, depending on the individual and the condition's severity.

Vitamin A: 10,000–35,000 IU
(Caution: megadoses of Vitamin A can be toxic. Don't take more than 10,000 IU without the advice of your health care professional; or use beta-carotene, a water-soluble precursor of vitamin A)

Vitamin B6: 10–200 mg

Vitamin B12: 10–1,000 mcg

Pantothenic acid: 50–1,000 mg

Riboflavin: 10–50 mg

Thiamine: 10–200 mg

Vitamin E: 100–1,000 IU

Iron: 20–50 mg.

Folic acid: 400–2,000 mcg

Copper: 2–4 mg

40

Herbal Healing

The common weed yellow dock remains one of the most common herbal alternatives for treating iron deficiency and iron-deficient anemia. The herb may work by enhancing the uptake of iron in the small intestine. However, if you take yellow dock by itself, the taste is so bitter you will probably want to use it in pill or tincture form.

If your anemia or blood deficiency does not respond to yellow dock, try increasing iron assimilation with stimulating digestive herbs such as gentian, burdock root, and dandelion root or leaves. In China, a number of digestion-enhancing herbs are thought to support the blood-building process. These include atractylodes, poria cocos (also known as hoelen fungus and *fu ling*), and ginger. Common Western spices, such as anise, caraway, cumin, mint, licorice, and linden flowers, can do the same.

Traditional Chinese Medicine treats blood deficiency with dong quai, white peony, and prepared rehmannia. These herbs are included in many traditional formulas to treat weak blood. Western herbalists also recommend several chlorophyll-rich herbs such as nettles, parsley, alfalfa, and watercress, taken as a tea or a concentrated powdered extract in capsules or tablets. The recipe below will give you a good start on rebuilding strong blood.

Iron Tea

1 teaspoon yellow dock root
1 teaspoon nettle leaves
1/2 teaspoon dandelion root
1/2 teaspoon beet greens
1/2 teaspoon licorice root
1 small piece cooked rehmannia root, if available
4 cups water

Bring herbs and water to a boil, then turn down the heat to a light simmer for 20 minutes. Turn off the heat and let steep another 20 minutes. Strain out the herbs. Drink 2 cups per day, one in the morning and one in the evening, around mealtimes. This formula can also be found as a tincture or in tablets or capsules of extracts.

CHAPTER 4

MOOD DISORDERS

One woman in ten experiences depression. Natural healing methods can support the therapies that help resolve it, and in some cases, replace common drug therapies.

Every woman feels blue once in a while. When a friend forgets to call, an accomplishment is slighted, or exhaustion sets in during the rush to finish a challenging project or meet family needs, anyone can feel low. Every life has these moments, but when feelings of grief, guilt, or hopelessness continue day after day or prevent enjoyment of usually satisfying activities, the problem may be clinical depression.

Just as every woman endures periods of sadness, she also occasionally experiences anxiety. After drinking an extra cup of coffee, or before a test or job interview, the anxiety may be simple nervousness or alertness. At other times—when a child bolts in front of the car, for instance—anxiety causes suddenly increased heart rate, shortness of breath, even dizziness or nausea. Those who speak or perform in public often report sweaty hands, dry mouth, and limbs that feel like they belong to someone else.

These symptoms are related to the "fight or flight" response that has aided human survival since ancient times. During emergencies, the body releases spurts of adrenaline and other chemicals that direct blood and energy to the muscles. These chemicals help the mind and nervous system take in more data and respond to crises quickly.

When this survival mechanism is used frequently, however, it takes a toll. The shaky, weak feeling that so often follows narrowly avoiding an accident is natural. After a nerve-wracking semester at school or a tempestuous romance, the body may require several weeks to rebuild energy. When daily commutes, work, or relationships are

St. John's wort

constantly stressful and anxiety-producing, physical, mental, and emotional health can break down and produce a continually anxious state.

Both anxiety and depression can result in insomnia—and be exacerbated by it. When it's 3 A.M. and you're turning over for the umpteenth time—with only another three hours to go before another fast and furious day—who can avoid feeling even more anxious? Even without anxiety or depression, women can have difficulty sleeping; physical, emotional, or hormonal changes—along with aging, poor diet, or bad sleeping habits—can conspire to deprive women of needed rest.

Luckily for women, herbal remedies for depression, anxiety, and insomnia are diverse, plentiful, effective, and safe—and often less expensive than pharmaceutical alternatives. For those with mild to moderate depression studies of St. John's wort's effectiveness compared to tricyclic antidepressants, or MAO inhibitors, have made headlines far beyond health journals. Because prescription antidepressants can have unwanted side effects and high prices, many conventional health professionals are now more open to alternative therapies.

DEPRESSION

In medical terms, depression is a mood disorder—a condition in which a continuing disturbance of mood becomes a central fact of life. Major depression is biochemical; in the acute phase, simple talk is of little use. Extreme symptoms that include slowed or agitated movement, too much or too little sleep, unwanted weight loss or gain, unwarranted guilt, and loss of pleasure in once-favorite activities indicate that professional help, preferably from a psychiatrist, is necessary. Untreated depression can lead to suicide. The line between "the blues" and depression that has taken on a life of its own is unclear, but those suffering sadness or bereavement typically don't feel worthless, hopeless, or full of self-doubt. When the depression is too intense, continues too long, and/or disrupts normal daily functions, the sufferer needs help.

How Many Sufferers?

Some surveys find that up to 20 percent of respondents report symptoms of depression. Studies typically show that 3 to 10 percent of the population experience mild or moderate depression as defined by the most widely accepted handbook of psychiatric symptoms and identification of disorders, the *Diagnostic and Statistical Manual of Mental Disorders* (DSM). Perhaps another 10 percent have some symptoms. Yet few who are afflicted by depression seek help.

Women are twice as likely to have symptoms of depression than men; one woman in ten experiences depression. Psychiatrists and researchers have theorized numerous reasons for this, focusing on biochemical and monthly hormone changes that result in reduced levels of serotonin, a neurotransmitter often associated with depression and insomnia. Women also can experience wider swings in thyroid function, and when thyroid levels are low, mood is typically low, too. Oral contraceptives and hormone replacement therapies contain estrogen that affects mood, too.

One theory why women suffer more depression proposes that during the process of development, a woman's sense of worth and value is strongly associated with her relationships with other people. Our society typically values these traits less than technical skills, leaving some women feeling frustrated and powerless. In turn, fear of disrupted relationships may lead women to "stuff" their feelings of frustration and powerlessness. They may turn their anger inward, blaming themselves for society's unwillingness to reward them. Conversely, as society opens opportunities to women, the pressure to achieve can also create stress, anxiety, and frustration.

Yet women have at least one advantage: their willingness to change, adapt, ask for help, and explore new ways of healing. During the many years we have been teaching herbal and natural-healing classes in various parts of the world, three times as many women as men typically

How to Know When You Need Help

How can you tell whether you're feeling a passing sadness or emotions for which you should seek help right away? You may feel fine around other people or at work but be immobilized by grief in other situations—or vice versa. It can be very difficult to objectively assess your own situation, especially when you are depressed or under stress. Help is seldom more than a telephone call away.

Your employer may have an Employee Assistance Program—a free, confidential counseling service to help you determine what kind of professional help you need; many health-insurance policies cover part or all of the cost of therapy. Many hospitals, universities, and colleges have crisis lines staffed by professionals or trained volunteers who can talk depression sufferers through a rough time or make an appointment for an evaluation. Sometimes help is available from a local church, spiritual organization, or women's center. If you feel your depression or anxiety has reached a level where you could injure yourself or someone else, do not isolate yourself. Pick up the phone and seek help.

attend. Women are more often willing to embrace new ways of healing and personal transformation.

What a Doctor Will Do

Just as there are many levels of depression and anxiety, there are many levels of treatment. After an initial screening, you and the professionals you consult may determine that you can best benefit by seeing a family or marriage counselor or a licensed social worker. Or you may be advised to have a complete evaluation from a psychiatrist, who will examine your physical, mental, and emotional health.

Your personal doctor can refer you to a psychiatrist; some insurance companies will require a referral before covering the expense. Through examination, interviews, and laboratory tests, the evaluation will determine whether you have clinical depression, and if so, what type. It may also determine whether your symptoms have a physical cause.

The interviewer will ask about your symptoms, how long you've had them, whether you've received treatment for depression in the past, and if so, what treatment. You also will be asked about alcohol or drug use and if you have had thoughts about suicide or death. A mental status test will determine whether your memory, speech, or thinking processes have been affected.

The chart on the next page, adapted from the DSM-IV, lists symptoms used to diagnose major depression. If you have five or more of these symptoms, seek psychiatric help immediately.

If you have less than five of these symptoms, but do not have them daily, you may be experiencing periods of mild to moderate depression. In this case, a psychiatrist or therapist, spiritual counselor, or health coach may be able to support your efforts to improve your overall outlook. The healing touch of a caring and skilled massage therapist also can work wonders. Acupuncture, herbal medicine, diet therapy and awareness, and physical activity all have great potential for healing mild, moderate, or severe depression or anxiety.

If you see a psychiatrist, he or she will prescribe psychotherapy, pharmaceutical drugs, or both. Although psychotherapy takes time and commitment, it aids in coping with stress and reducing anxiety and addresses the root of the problem.

Therapies for depression vary. Exploration therapy encourages patients to explore unresolved inner conflicts. Becoming aware of unhealthy thoughts and deliberately replacing them with more positive ones is often an important part of the exploration process. Behavioral therapy uses a system of rewards and punishments to reinforce positive, healthy behavior. Relaxation training involves teaching deep relaxation methods for mastering anxiety; techniques may include progressive muscle relaxation, biofeedback training, guided imagery, and visualization. These techniques can be of great help not only in reducing anxiety but also in helping the body adjust to a change of habits, such as quitting smoking or eliminating unhealthy foods.

An Overview of Antidepressant Drugs

In cases of persistent chronic depression or an acute episode of depression, physicians or psychiatrists are likely to prescribe medication.

In the last ten years, powerful drugs have been developed that change the balance of neurotransmitters, the substances that allow nerve

CRITERIA FOR A MAJOR DEPRESSIVE EPISODE

Five or more of the following symptoms have been present during the same two-week period and represent a change from previous functioning. At least one symptom must be either item 1 or item 2 on the list.

1. Depressed mood most of the day, nearly every day.

2. Noticeably reduced interest or pleasure in all or many activities most of the day, nearly every day.

3. Significant unwanted weight loss or weight gain.

4. Insomnia or abnormal wakefulness nearly every night.

5. Feelings of agitation or anxiety, self-assessed or noticed by others.

6. Fatigue or loss of energy nearly every day.

7. Feelings of worthlessness or excessive or inappropriate guilt nearly every day.

8. Diminished ability to think or concentrate, or indecisiveness, nearly every day, self-assessed or noticed by others.

9. Recurrent thoughts of death or suicide.

10. Clinically significant distress or impairment in social, occupational, or other important areas of functioning.

11. Symptoms are not due to the direct physical effects of a substance such as prescription or recreational drugs or a general medical condition like hypothyroidism.

12. Symptoms are not accounted for by grief after loss of a loved one.

Source: Modified from DSM-IV.

impulses to travel in the brain and nervous system. The newest are SSRIs—selective serotonin reuptake inhibitors—known by the trade names Prozac, Paxil, or Zoloft. These drugs can be extremely helpful for some patients. The choice of SSRI depends on many factors, such as other medications and individual biochemistry.

SSRIs not only improve mood but can be used to reduce mental dwelling—that "can't get it off my mind" feeling—thereby providing tremendous relief for certain types of anxiety, such as obsessive-compulsive disorder. Although Zoloft, Paxil, and Prozac cost more than older antidepressants, they usually have fewer side effects. The mildest include nausea and headache, which usually disappear as the body adjusts to the medication. About 25 percent of those taking SSRIs experience impaired sexuality, reporting decreased libido and failed orgasm. Side effects that fade with continued use include anxiety, agitation, insomnia, and unwanted weight change. The drugs are not effective for everyone.

Before Prozac and its cousins became available, mood-changing drugs were limited to tricyclic or heterocyclic antidepressants (TCAs), including Elavil, Imipramine, and Desipramine. Although these antidepressants are cheaper than SSRIs, their drawbacks can be severe. Adverse effects include sleepiness, tremors, blurred vision, possible aggravation of psychosis, weight gain, and withdrawal symptoms. TCAs are also very dangerous in cases of overdose. This is a concern because depressed patients are often prone to suicide attempts. An overdose of these drugs can cause coma, respiratory depression, seizures, and heart-rhythm abnormalities.

Another class of antidepressants, the monoamine oxidase inhibitors (MAOIs) includes Parnate and Nardil. These are usually reserved as backup drugs because they can cause very serious interactions with foods and other drugs. When combined with foods containing tyramine, including wine and some cheeses, MAOIs cause blood pressure to shoot up. The MAOIs can also severely interact with SSRIs to cause serotonin syndrome, a condition characterized by hyperthermia, muscle rigidity, and changes in mental status. Other side effects of MAOIs include headache, drowsiness, dry mouth, and weight gain, but overdoses are rare.

The use of all these drugs requires careful monitoring by a physician, or psychiatrist.

Newer Antidepressants

In recent years, drug companies have sought to develop new antidepressants that relieve depression as well as SSRIs, but without the side effects. So far, none has been entirely successful.

Welbutrin (bupropion hydrochloride) eases depression without affecting sexuality, but it often induces nervousness and insomnia. Welbutrin also slightly increases risk of seizure. Serzone (nefazodone hydrochloride) has been gaining in popularity, although it can interact with MAOIs to cause severe reactions. Effexor (venlafaxine hydrochloride) can result in nausea and sedation, and Remeron (mirtazapine) can be sedating while causing moderate weight gain. If you change doctors, be certain that your new health-care professional knows the complete history of what has been prescribed for you.

ANXIETY

Like depression, anxiety can have a physical cause such as thyroid imbalance or alcohol withdrawal. Treating the physical disorder may reduce or eliminate some anxiety. Sometimes the cause is purely emotional: stress from work or relationship difficulties. Sometimes counseling alone may be successful; for some severe cases of anxiety, doctors may recommend a combination of psychotherapy, relaxation training, and medication.

What a Doctor Will Do

To treat severe anxiety doctors often prescribe three main types of medication: the SSRIs used to treat depression (Prozac, Paxil, and Zoloft); the sedative benzodiazepines, such as Valium, Xanax, Ativan, and Librium; and BuSpar, or buspirone hydrochloride.

Valium and similar drugs can relieve the physical symptoms of anxiety within an hour, but they are extremely addicting and can have serious side effects such as memory loss and mental confusion. They are best taken in extreme cases and only for short periods. BuSpar, a relatively new drug, can reduce anxiety without addiction for some.

TAKING CONTROL OF YOUR MEDICATIONS

Although the exact mechanisms of antidepressants are unknown, their classification can be useful. If a particular SSRI gives you serious side effects, ask your doctor to prescribe one from another group. However, interactions between the different groups of antidepressants can be severe. A physician or psychiatrist must supervise changing from one medication to another.

In addition, a new antidepressant may offer you no relief or benefits that fade after several months. Why? So many factors influence depression and other mood disorders that no one drug or treatment works for everyone. For some, even a combination of drugs is useless. What's most important is following your instincts about what works and what doesn't, and working with your health-care practitioner to change strategies if one doesn't seem to be effective. Be patient; antidepressants can take up to a week or two to show results. An adequate period is four to six weeks.

INSOMNIA

You don't need a doctor to tell you your sleep is disrupted, but you may need one to tell you why. Insomnia can arise from an undetected physical condition, upsets in biological rhythm such as a new work schedule, stimulating foods like coffee, or sensitivity to medicines. Women sometimes experience insomnia as part of premenstrual syndrome or while approaching menopause when hormone levels fluctuate. Those with endometriosis may experience insomnia before and until the cessation of menstruation.

Many women experience insomnia when dealing with specific emotional or personal issues. The loss of a loved one, a divorce, or a problem at work can create emotional, mental, and physical stress that easily disrupts sleep, even when it does not result in symptoms of anxiety or depression. Environmental factors, even subtle ones, can contribute to disrupted sleep. We all know what that's like—loud, sudden noises, bright lights—you name it, we're awake.

What a Doctor Will Do

The majority of people buy over-the-counter medications that contain sedative-type antihistamines. These drugs—Unisom, Sominex, Nytol, Sleep-Eze and similar products—may help with mild or occasional sleeplessness, but they are not recommended for prolonged use because they can be habit-forming.

The same benzodiazepines used for anxiety may be used for insomnia. They are extremely effective for inducing sleep, reducing the amount of time it takes to fall asleep, and the number of times the sleeper awakens during the night. Nonetheless, benzodiazepines are powerfully addictive drugs that should not be used except under a doctor's care and they should *never* be discontinued without a doctor's supervision. Further, they reduce the quality of sleep and often leave a "hangover" the next day. Most doctors prescribe them for acute bouts of insomnia, to be used at the lowest dose for only a few days.

Psychotherapy for Depression, Anxiety, and Insomnia

Psychotherapy can be effective in treating depression, anxiety, and any resulting insomnia, whether used alone or combined with drug therapy. Psychotherapy involves regular meetings between an individual and the therapist. Once goals are established, a patient may discuss her current problems and stressors as well as her past. The therapy may focus on problem-solving skills, overcoming inappropriate thought patterns, or healing emotional wounds. Psychotherapy may last for only a few meetings or continue for months.

A key factor in psychotherapy's success is the individual's trust in and alliance with the therapist. To help find a good fit for therapy, talk to friends and get referrals. Speaking briefly on the phone with several therapists may help you find one with a natural rapport.

NATURAL HEALING

Whether a doctor prescribes antidepressants, psychotherapy, both or neither, there are many effective natural healing strategies for depression, anxiety, and insomnia. Some may be as basic as changing habits connected with when you sleep and how. Changes in diet can have a surprising effect on mood. Aromatherapists know of many scents that may have a mood-lifting effect. And just about everyone has heard that the herb St. John's wort helps many cases of mild to moderate depression. It's only one of many natural remedies that can assist in easing anxiety, promoting sleep, and healing mood disorders.

Healthy Habits

To cope with mild anxiety, many find friendly assurances, a soothing touch, and a safe environment effective. We have found that vigorous exercise is one of the best anxiety-releasing medicines available. When energy builds up in muscles, it becomes tension. Tension impedes the free flow of blood-borne nutrients and oxygen, vital energy, hormones, and nerve substances. How can the body work properly under these circumstances?

For more persistent or stronger anxiety, add daily relaxation techniques such as biofeedback, meditation, visualization, and deep breathing. We highly recommend yoga, tai chi, or qi gong, all of which regulate vital energy and release tension.

Dietary Changes

In our experience, increasing protein intake probably influences mood more than any other dietary change. Vegetarians who eat fewer than 70 grams of protein daily or those who eat meat only once or twice a week may benefit from more protein. If this is your situation, try eating fish, chicken, or vegetable sources of protein up to four times a week, or even daily. Daily intake of red meat, however, irritates the nervous system; eat it only once or twice a week.

Why does adding protein relieve mood problems? Protein foods contain amino acids, some of which are crucial to the brain's chemistry. L-tryptophan, for example, is the precursor to the important neurotransmitter serotonin. Although doctors can prescribe L-tryptophan, it is difficult to obtain. Fortunately, this amino acid is found in high concentrations in a number of foods such as spirulina, almonds, nutritional yeast, and chicken.

Serotonin and other neurotransmitters are integral to modulating nerve function. The table below summarizes the important amino acids that have been shown to help with depression, anxiety and insomnia, and the foods that contain them. Some amino acids are also available in natural products stores in their pure form, but beware of supplementing your diet with pure amino acids for extended periods, which may create an imbalance.

Other Foods to Add

Nearly everyone today can benefit from adding more vegetables to the diet, especially dark, leafy greens. Depression, anxiety, and stress can take a toll on the adrenal glands, the digestive system, and liver, as do some of the prescription drugs used to relieve these conditions.

AMINO ACIDS HELPFUL IN MOOD DISORDERS

Amino Acid	Food Sources	Action	Uses
Glycine	Turkey, wheat germ, carrots, cottage cheese, celery, almonds	Sedative	Eases depression
Isoleucine	Wheat germ, olives, avocados, cheese, yogurt, chicken, almonds, walnuts	Acts as a neurotransmitter	Encourages appetite, protects against stress
Tryptophan	Spirulina; nutritional yeast; soy, pinto and mung beans; tempeh; tofu; lentils; fish; chicken	Precursor of serotonin	Reduces pain, insomnia, depression, and other mood disorders, appetite imbalances
Valine	Wheat germ, almonds, carrots, cheese, yogurt, chicken, apples	Acts as a neurotransmitter	Encourages appetite, protects against stress

Source: Braverman, 1987

Whether or not your healing program includes these drugs, you may want to adjust your diet to focus on foods that support and tone these organs and systems.

Adding grains such as basmati or brown rice and millet over a period of several weeks or months may produce a calming and relaxing effect on the liver and thus on your emotions. Beans are especially grounding and supportive to the adrenal system. To prepare adzuki, mung, and other small beans, soak them overnight before cooking, replacing the water at least twice, then cook until tender. Adding several tablespoons of whole sea vegetables such as nori or wakame adds flavor, texture, and nutrients. Winter squash, yams, and root vegetables such as carrots and burdock (gobo) support the body's hormones. Almonds, which are high in tryptophan, are easily added to cereals, casseroles, stir-fries, and other dishes. You can also make your own almond milk and drink it warm at bedtime to foster relaxed sleep.

Problem Foods: Sugar and Stimulants

Foods containing simple sugars and artificial stimulants increase metabolism. For those with rapid metabolisms, the blood-sugar roller-coaster experienced after eating sweets can exacerbate mood swings. In Traditional Chinese Medicine, these foods are thought to deplete vital energy. The lack of this life force, or Qi, is likely to be a major cause of depression.

Limiting simple sugars to fresh fruit in season can help stabilize mood swings and allow a steadier release of energy, but this is certainly more

Almond Milk

Almond milk is available at health food stores, but it is easy and inexpensive to make at home. If you suffer from insomnia, try a warm cup of almond milk before bed.

1 cup of organic (if available) almonds
1 quart of water
Vanilla to taste (optional)

Soak almonds in water overnight. In the morning, blend almonds and water at high speed until smooth and creamy. Add a little vanilla if you wish. Store in the refrigerator but use quickly; it will ferment after a few days. Or you can soak the almonds overnight, drain, and then refrigerate, blending a little at a time. The almonds will last up to a week.

easily said than done. Sugar lurks in almost every packaged food, including condiments and salad dressings, and in supposedly healthy foods, such as some dried fruits and pasta sauces. Try gradually trimming sugar-rich foods and substituting fresh fruit—if necessary, temporarily add very small amounts of honey or maple syrup.

Anxiety and insomnia sufferers may also benefit from limiting or eliminating caffeine; during times of extreme stress, it's easy to increase your caffeine intake without noticing. Coffee, black tea, cola drinks, and chocolate are common caffeine sources. Caffeine causes dependency, so reduce it gradually and in consultation with your health-care provider, especially if you are taking drug therapy. Caffeine and other stimulants can also be problematic for depression sufferers, because the stimulants mask symptoms while allowing the root causes to go unaddressed.

SUPPLEMENTS FOR DEPRESSION, ANXIETY, AND INSOMNIA

Vitamin E: 400 IU

B complex: niacin, pantothenic acid, riboflavin, vitamin B6, folic acid

Spirulina, 1 teaspoon or 4 capsules or tablets, morning and evening

Calcium and magnesium: about 1200 mg of magnesium, 800 mg of calcium a day.

Dietary Supplements

Vitamin deficiencies associated with depression include biotin, calcium, copper, iron, folic acid, niacin, pantothenic acid, potassium, pyridoxine, thiamine, Vitamin C, and B12. The best strategy may be to add a good nutritional-system product containing sea vegetables, spirulina, and herb extracts to the diet. The B vitamins are especially important for anxiety patients, who may benefit from a well-balanced B-complex supplement or the addition of 1 tablespoon of nutritional yeast to each meal.

Herbal Healing

Herbs offer a strong arsenal for fighting depression, anxiety, and insomnia. Nearly everyone knows that St. John's wort helps many depression sufferers, but newcomers to herbal medicine may not know about the host of other herbs that can assist this powerful plant to lift mood and promote helpful sleep. Like St. John's wort, these herbs have few if any side effects. Other herbal formulas, known as constitutional remedies, can help repair body systems damaged by long-term depression or anxiety attacks.

St. John's wort, a yellow-flowering perennial, is the premier herbal remedy for depression. It should be used with caution if you take antidepressant drugs because there is a possibility that it interacts with some antidepressants. The recommended dose of the dark-red tincture or liquid extract is one-half to 1 teaspoon (2.5 to 5 ml) twice daily. Standardized extracts of St. John's wort are also available in capsules or tablets; take two in the morning and one in the evening.

Most women who take St. John's wort extract find that the effects take two to three weeks to fully develop. If you are now taking an antidepressant and wish to switch to St. John's wort, work with your doctor and possibly with a qualified herbal practitioner to make the transition. As an antidepressant, St. John's wort usually takes about two months to reach full effectiveness. For some types of chronic insomnia, a low to moderate dose, continued for several months, can help. There are some indications that St. John's wort may increase sensitivity to sunlight when taken in large doses over time, especially if you are fair-skinned with blue eyes.

Calming Herbs: The Relaxing Trio

Valerian, California poppy, and kava kava can work wonders for jangled nerves and help ease insomnia and anxiety. Because depression is often accompanied by insomnia, anxiety, or both, many formulas for depression include calming herbs. Each of the trio has a slightly different action in the body.

MELATONIN "MAGIC"

Melatonin is a hormone secreted by the pineal gland and associated with the body's internal clock, which governs the biological cycles of waking and sleep. When taken as a supplement, melatonin can work wonders for some, but others get no results or even experience side effects. St. John's wort can increase the body's natural level of melatonin.

Leading researchers are unsure how melatonin affects the body or how safe it is, especially for long-term use, but melatonin provides a natural and peaceful sleep, with ample periods of the most restorative phase of sleep. It may best be used on a short-term basis. The average daily dose of melatonin is 3 mg, although individual dosages vary. Common side effects include grogginess, tiredness, headaches, and depression. Long-term use may lead to nightmares and lowered sex drive. Children and teens should not take it.

Consult a health practitioner before using melatonin if you are pregnant or nursing; or if you suffer from serious illness such as autoimmune disease, leukemia, lymphoma, diabetes, hormone imbalance, or depression; or if you are using antidepressants or medications that suppress immune function.

Antidepressant Tincture

This formula combines St. John's wort with kava kava, two types of ginseng, and reishi, which strengthens immunity and regulates estrogen.

1 teaspoon St. John's wort tincture
1/2 teaspoon kava kava root tincture
1/2 teaspoon American ginseng tincture
1/2 teaspoon Siberian ginseng (eleuthero) tincture
1/2 teaspoon reishi extract (substitute tincture of hawthorn leaf
and flower if necessary)

Combine tinctures in a dark glass bottle. Take 2 droppersful, 3 times daily; up to 8 droppersful daily can be taken during a crisis. To avoid alcohol, purchase glycerin tinctures instead, or take the herbs in the same proportion in pills or as a strong tea.

Valerian is an excellent herbal sedative that has none of the negative side effects of Valium or other synthetic sedatives. It combines well with other calming herbs, such as California poppy, skullcap, hops, and passion flower. Valerian helps bring on sleep, especially among the elderly or habitually poor sleepers, and even confirmed insomniacs report benefit from the herb. Valerian and California poppy are both useful when one is withdrawing from antianxiety drugs such as Valium. (Despite similar names, the herb valerian and the pharmaceutical Valium bear no resemblance to one another, either in results or in chemistry.)

California poppy is also very effective against nervousness, sleeplessness, and anxiety. It blends well with valerian, passion flower, and other calming herbs and can be used as tincture, capsules, or tablets. California poppy can be found in a number of commercial preparations. It is non-narcotic and cannot affect tests for illegal drugs.

Kava kava, taken before bedtime, helps relax muscles and promote sleep. Some people get great results. Many new extracts of kava kava are becoming available in natural products stores and even drug stores. Try a different brand if you don't find it effective, because all extracts are not created equal.

Reishi is an ancient Chinese herb that is believed to calm the spirit and nourish the heart. In Traditional Chinese Medicine, the heart system relates to emotional and mental poise. Take two or three capsules or tablets of reishi extract for several months for full benefit. Popular Chinese herbal patent formulas for sleeping problems include An Mien Pan, Ping Xin Wan, Bu Xin Don, and Xiao Yao Wan; these are often available in natural product and herb stores.

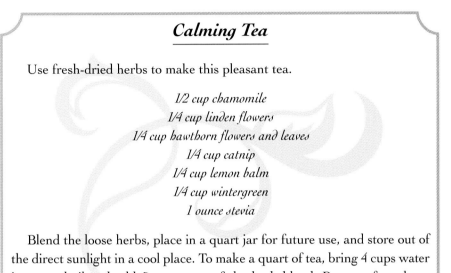

Calming Tea

Use fresh-dried herbs to make this pleasant tea.

1/2 cup chamomile
1/4 cup linden flowers
1/4 cup hawthorn flowers and leaves
1/4 cup catnip
1/4 cup lemon balm
1/4 cup wintergreen
1 ounce stevia

Blend the loose herbs, place in a quart jar for future use, and store out of the direct sunlight in a cool place. To make a quart of tea, bring 4 cups water just to a boil and add 5 teaspoons of the herb blend. Remove from heat, cover, and let steep for 20 minutes. Strain, reheat if necessary, and drink, or refrigerate for up to three days. Drink several cups daily or before bedtime as needed.

Calming Herbal Extract

3 teaspoons California poppy tincture
2½ teaspoons hawthorn tincture
2 teaspoons valerian tincture
1½ teaspoons kava kava tincture
1 teaspoon reishi tincture

Combine all ingredients. Take 1 teaspoon of the tincture two or three times daily. If desired, substitute the same proportions of capsules or tablets.

Constitutional Support

In Traditional Chinese Medicine, fundamental imbalances in the body are thought to be the root of depression, anxiety, and insomnia. Several body systems can benefit from additional support during the healing process: the liver, the adrenals, and the digestive systems.

During emotional healing, pay attention to the liver; TCM teaches that the health of the liver brings health and balance to the emotions. Liver cleansers such as roots of dandelion, burdock, or yellow dock help the liver produce bile, which in turn rids the body of toxins. If you abuse alcohol or drugs or you are weaning yourself from antidepressants, look for herbal formulas that support the liver, such as milk thistle, the common spices turmeric and ginger, and dandelion and burdock root.

The adrenal glands, located atop the kidneys, react to stress or the threat of danger by producing adrenaline and additional hormones that regulate immune function. When stress or anxiety disorders continually activate these glands, the immune system can become depleted and the digestive tract impaired. If you are generally fatigued, yet have sleeping disorders, look for herbal support formulas that contain one or more of the herbs rehmannia, Siberian ginseng (eleuthero), American ginseng, Chinese wild yam, kudzu, reishi, schisandra, or licorice root.

Finally, chronic stress and anxiety almost always affect the digestive system. Try increasing nutrient absorption with yellow dock root or a bitters preparation containing such herbs as gentian, ginger, angelica, cardamom, artichoke leaf, or orange peel. Chinese herbs thought to build strong digestion include atractylodes, poria, and ginger.

Bedtime Tea

This tried-and-true formula is a very effective sleep-inducer. You can measure the herbs by weight or by volume so long as the proportions remain the same.

3 ounces valerian
2 ounces linden flowers
2 ounces kava kava
2 ounces chamomile
1 ounce catnip

Blend the herbs together and store in a tightly sealed jar away from light. Make a tea by bringing water just to a boil and steeping 1 teaspoon to 1 tablespoon of herbs per cup for 20 minutes. Strain and drink up to 1 cup before bed, sweetened with a little honey, licorice, or stevia if you wish.

Adrenal/Hormonal Toner

1 teaspoon reishi tincture
1 teaspoon valerian tincture
1/2 teaspoon rehmannia tincture
1/2 teaspoon American ginseng tincture
1/2 teaspoon orange peel tincture

Blend the tinctures together and take 1 teaspoon in a little water, 2 to 3 times daily. Take one dose before bedtime. A tea is also effective.

Harmonious Mood Elixir

1 teaspoon California poppy tincture
1 teaspoon St. John's wort tincture
1 teaspoon American ginseng tincture
1 teaspoon honey, glycerin, stevia extract or licorice extract
3 to 5 drops essential oil of orange

Blend the tinctures together. Take as needed during emergencies, up to one teaspoon every few hours. Otherwise, take one teaspoon twice daily as a general relaxing aid.

Insomnia Tincture

Strange surroundings often result in short-term insomnia. This tincture travels more easily than a tea, although you can combine the dried herbs in the same proportions.

1/2 teaspoon valerian tincture
1/2 teaspoon hops tincture
1/2 teaspoon passion flower tincture
1/2 teaspoon chamomile tincture

Blend ingredients. Take 2 or 3 teaspoons half an hour before bed.

Aromatherapy

Although aromatherapy alone isn't completely effective against mood disorders, it makes a safe adjunct treatment when combined with herbal and pharmaceutical antidepressants. For a simple case of the blues, it's very useful. Scent impressions go directly to the brain, where they are thought to adjust brain chemistry.

Some of the most often-used mood-lifting essential oils are the citrus fragrances—orange peel, grapefruit, and orange blossom (also known as neroli). Lavender and chamomile are excellent individually or in blends. Add a few drops of an appealing aroma to a bath or a massage oil; scent the room with it if you wish. Carry a small vial of a calming essential oil with you and simply take a whiff when you feel your anxiety level rise.

Sleep-inducing scents are plentiful. A few drops of lavender essential oil added to a foot bath or regular bath can have a nice, calming effect. Sleep pillows made of hops, lavender, and chamomile and bath salts containing relaxing essential oils are available in many natural products stores. It's easy to make your own sleep pillow.

Hops Sleep Pillow

1/4 cup dried hops strobiles
1/8 cup dried chamomile flowers
1/8 cup dried lavender flowers (optional)
2 pieces of fabric about 8 inches square

Sew right sides of fabric together around all four edges, leaving an opening large enough to insert a tablespoon. Turn right side out. Combine herbs and spoon them into the pillow. Sew the opening closed by hand. Lay the hops pillow under your regular sleeping pillow. If you are feeling creative, you can make the pillow in any shape or size. Just make more of this herb blend to fill it.

CHAPTER 5

MENSTRUATION

*Five days of pain or a simple, symptomless monthly event?
Every woman's period is different. For many women, herbs can help
ease menstrual symptoms.*

Menstruation is a normal part of life for healthy women of reproductive age, but every woman experiences her period differently. The menstrual flow of some is painless and as predictable as clockwork; other women experience low back pain, nausea, and severe, incapacitating cramps. Some women lose very little blood—less than two ounces—but others bleed enough to bring on anemia, fatigue, and dizziness. Other common symptoms can include thigh pain, sweating, and headaches.

Physical conditions, not mental illness or imagination, cause most menstrual difficulties. Hormone imbalances, endometriosis, uterine infection, fibroid cysts, scar tissue, or a troublesome IUD may be involved. Anatomical problems, such as a tilted uterus, are occasionally at fault. Stress and emotional upsets, especially when intense and prolonged, can also affect menstrual symptoms.

Normal menstruation occurs in a three-part cycle governed by the body's hormonal signals. In the first part of the cycle, the uterine lining, or the outer layer of the endometrium, is shed during menstruation. Then the endometrium and its blood vessels and glands regrow, becoming dense with capillaries, in anticipation of possible pregnancy. After one of the ovaries releases a mature egg, ready to be fertilized, the endometrium's blood vessels undergo changes that allow them to deliver more blood. The glands of the endometrium begin to secrete mucus. If a fertilized egg does not implant itself in this spongy medium by about six to eight days after ovulation, the uterine lining breaks down and drains from the uterus through the vagina. Then the cycle begins anew,

Cramp bark

orchestrated by the complex interaction between hormones. This process sounds straightforward—but for many women who suffer from menstrual difficulties, it is neither simple nor painless.

Painful Menstruation

Prostaglandins, hormone-like substances, are thought to be the culprits behind menstrual cramps. These substances, which are responsible for regulating smooth-muscle activity, can cause uterine contractions and decrease blood flow to the uterus. Prostaglandins signal the uterus to empty during menstruation and contract during childbirth.

> ### RISK FACTORS FOR MENSTRUAL PAIN
>
> Young age at onset of menstruation
>
> Long menstrual periods
>
> Smoking cigarettes
>
> Being overweight

Brief, mild cramping during the early days of the period usually is normal; the uterus typically contracts to some degree to expel the uterine lining. High levels of certain prostaglandins can cause excessive uterine contractions that result in pain. Discomfort can also result when these substances decrease blood flow to the uterus, because metabolic by-products can build up in the tissues.

The drop in levels of calcium and magnesium during menstruation may be another factor in cramps; both of these minerals help muscles relax and repair.

What a Doctor Will Do

Modern medicine classifies dysmenorrhea, or painful periods, into two types, primary and secondary. When no physical abnormality or disease process causes painful menstruation, it is called primary dysmenorrhea. When a condition such as fibroids or endometriosis causes or is related to the pain, doctors describe it as secondary amenorrhea.

Usually, doctors will first try prescribing anti-inflammatory pain relievers such as aspirin, ibuprofen (Motrin, Advil), naproxen (Naprosyn), mefenamic acid (Ponstel), and other nonsteroidal anti-inflammatory drugs (NSAIDs). These drugs inhibit prostaglandin synthesis. They are successful up to 80 percent of the time when taken at the onset of pain and continued until it ends.

Like most pain-relieving drugs, NSAIDs are processed by the liver and stress that organ; we recommend caution in using these drugs if you have liver disease or drink alcohol regularly. Some NSAIDs produce side effects, including rebound headaches, gastrointestinal upset, and sometimes a feeling of "spaciness." Long-term use may lead to inflammation and ulcers of the digestive tract.

Another option for relieving painful menstruation, birth-control pills, is also about 80 percent effective. The hormones in the contraceptives inhibit ovulation and decrease the amount of uterine lining produced in a cycle. The long-term use of contraceptive hormones has been linked to increased risk of some cancers. Newer pill formulas that combine estrogen with progesterone increase risk of endometrial cancer and probably breast cancers by a much smaller amount, but long-term use still increases the risk of liver cancer and cardiovascular problems.

Some women also report feeling lethargic around the time of menstruation. These individuals should be checked for anemia, low blood sugar, and other conditions that diminish energy.

Excessive Bleeding

By lowering respiration and blood pressure, normal menstruation reduces a woman's level of physical energy only slightly. Heavy bleeding on a regular basis, however, can cause light-headedness, exhaustion, and anemia. Because excessive bleeding can signal problems such as endometriosis, be sure to investigate the cause.

Of course, the term "heavy bleeding" is subjective, because every woman's blood flow varies. The same volume of blood loss that may be normal for a large woman may cause anemia for a small or slightly-built one. Generally, if a woman has to change her pad or tampon every hour for seven days, she is losing enough blood that she should seek immediate medical attention. If her bleeding is heavy enough that she experiences light-headedness or fatigue that interferes with usual activities, she may want to consult a health-care practitioner.

Heavy menstrual periods can be blamed on a long list of conditions, most of them hormonal. Endometriosis, uterine fibroid cysts or infection, cancer, an ectopic pregnancy, an IUD, and blood-thinning drugs all may contribute to heavy menstruation. Other factors include vitamin A deficiency or liver imbalances. Stressful situations or prolonged emotional turmoil may disrupt hormones and cause more bleeding, as may the excessive use of drugs or alcohol.

What a Doctor Will Do

An examination to determine the cause of excessive bleeding should include a pelvic exam for the presence of fibroids, endometriosis, or other abnormalities. Blood tests should also be done to determine whether a blood disorder or anemia exists. Other tests may include endometrial sampling, various hormonal tests, or hysteroscopy, which entails examination of the interior of the uterus using a small lighted scope. For bleeding associated with clots or endometriosis, the overgrowth of tissue and resultant heavy bleeding often can be stopped by a D&C, or dilation of the cervix and curettage, in which the uterine lining is scraped away.

The primary medical treatment to stop excessive bleeding is contraceptive drugs, for five to seven days. Other hormonal treatments include other drugs that suppress ovarian function, such as Danazol, but they have numerous side effects, including the cessation of menstruation, and their dosages must be carefully adjusted for the individual. When excessive bleeding continues and drugs don't work, doctors may recommend hysterectomy, especially if the patient is beyond her childbearing years.

An examination to determine the cause of excessive bleeding should check for the presence of fibroids, endometriosis, or other abnormalities.

Irregular Menstruation

Menstruation usually follows ovulation like clockwork; a woman begins bleeding fourteen days after releasing an egg. Some women have slightly longer or shorter menstrual cycles; the most important thing is that the cycle be fairly regular. The exception is the approach of menopause, beginning in the late 40s and early 50s, when menstruation normally shortens and becomes irregular. Young teenagers also experience irregular menstrual cycles with some frequency.

About 80 percent of women whose cycles are irregular can track the problem to hormonal imbalances or disruptions. Additional symptoms may include sugar intolerance, anxiety, and depression.

In the remaining 20 percent of cases, a variety of conditions may be the cause, but they may be related to hormonal imbalance. Sporadic ovulation, for instance, may indicate too little or too much estrogen. A woman may need to switch her oral contraceptive formula. Either high or low amounts of thyroid hormones can trigger an irregular cycle.

If ovulation is taking place on schedule, the source of irregular menstrual periods could be a physical problem in the uterus, such as fibroids, endometriosis, a tumor, or adenomyosis, in which the uterine lining grows into the muscle tissue. Irregular bleeding can also be caused by prolonged emotional turmoil or excessive use of drugs or alcohol.

What a Doctor Will Do

Unless your irregular cycle is obviously due to stress, it may not be easy for you to figure out what is causing the problem. Get a pelvic exam to rule out a serious disorder. Doctors usually check levels of the major hormones as well as for pregnancy. An ultrasound can help determine if there are any growths or other abnormalities in the uterus.

If the irregularity involves bleeding mid-cycle, a doctor will check for tumors, fibroids, endometriosis, cancer, and hormonal imbalances. If the cycle is late, the first possibility may be pregnancy or disease. Once these have been ruled out, standard treatment is birth-control pills. While these are effective in making the cycle regular, they carry a risk for breast or endometrial cancer, depending on the type of hormones used.

Missing or Scanty Periods

Women who have reached puberty but haven't begun menstruating, or who began, but stopped, have amenorrhea. Scanty menstrual flow, or periods skipped for reasons other than pregnancy, is called oligomenorrhea. The underlying cause of both stopped periods and scanty periods is typically a failure of the hypothalamic, pituitary, and sex glands to work together to bring about menstruation.

Some women undoubtedly consider it a blessing *not* to menstruate. It's certainly more convenient! But cessation of menstrual periods can be a symptom of a problem that could have lasting effects on health (notably osteoporosis) and longevity, so it should not be ignored.

Sometimes the cause of missed or scanty periods is easy to pinpoint. High stress levels, withdrawal from birth-control pills, uterine surgery, or infection can disrupt menstruation, as may chemotherapy and radiation treatments. Extremely thin or very athletic women whose body fat percentage is extremely low may stop menstruating.

Dr. Tori Hudson, a naturopathic physician with extensive experience in women's health, suggests that emotions often play a role when a woman's well-established periods stop. Hudson often recommends that her patients seek counseling along with their other treatments.

Amenorrhea is divided into two classifications. Primary amenorrhea is diagnosed when a woman age 16 or older does not begin her periods. Chromosomal abnormality, hormonal imbalance, or glandular tumors often are the underlying cause; occasionally the hymen has no opening for the passage of menstrual flow. Drug or alcohol abuse can also cause amenorrhea; so can a thyroid imbalance, tumors of the ovaries, and pelvic inflammatory disease.

When menstruation stops for a minimum of three months in a woman with previously established periods, the condition is known as secondary amenorrhea. Chemotherapy, radiation treatments, anorexia nervosa, premature ovarian failure, various types of tumors, and hormonal imbalances may cause it. It's also not uncommon in women who are very athletic and do not produce enough estrogen.

What A Doctor Will Do

Examination to find the cause of these conditions includes evaluation of the breasts and vulva as well as an internal pelvic exam. Diagnostic tests may be ordered to measure the levels of estrogens, progesterones, and prolactins in the blood. But manipulating hormone levels is not an easy task. It may involve a good deal of experimentation to get the dosages of artificial hormones balanced to the patient's benefit, and the adjustment period may be difficult.

Natural Healing

While different types of menstrual problems have specific natural healing solutions, some general health recommendations apply to all.

Don't smoke. We can't say it often enough: If you do smoke cigarettes, one of the best things you can do for yourself is quit now. In addition to smoking's well-publicized health threats such as cancer, smoking also lowers oxygen intake. This increases painful menstrual cramps and can add depression, irritability, and headaches to menstrual problems. The British Birth Cohort study of 2,181 women showed that all of these problems are more common in young women who smoke than in others.

Monitor your stress level. Some cultures have long recognized the need of menstruating women for a little extra nurturing. For instance, some Native American women traditionally retreat from family responsibilities and relax in a menstrual or "moon" lodge every month. Of course, this custom would be difficult to translate to a hectic Western lifestyle. But if your periods are regular, you at least have the opportunity to plan some extra rest and relaxation at this time.

Normalize your exercise level. If you are generally sedentary, try to get more exercise, especially for your stomach and back muscles. But if you are an athlete and amenorrhea is a problem, you may want to re-evaluate your athletic training schedule and your caloric intake. Ask your doctor to refer you to an exercise physiologist or dietician.

Get some sunlight. Some research suggests that a woman's cycle may be partly regulated by light. Too much time spent under artificial lights and not enough real sunlight can change the cycle. Our bodies can also synthesize vitamin D from natural sunlight; the deficiency of this vitamin is implicated in some menstrual disorders.

Dietary Changes

Foods that may help reduce production of the prostaglandins that can cause cramps include spinach, beans, millet, alfalfa, mango, wheat germ oil, chia seeds, and purslane. Nettle greens and other green leafy vegetables are loaded with the muscle-relaxing minerals calcium and magnesium. You can also take flaxseed oil and increase your intake of raw seeds and nuts to boost beneficial fatty acids.

Stay away from fried foods such as potato and corn chips, crackers, baked goods, and anything that contains hydrogenated oils, including margarine. This processed oil may disrupt the body's metabolism of fatty acids and reduce the amount of oxygen in the cells. Drinking alcohol or eating eggs, meat, and dairy foods may increase menstrual cramps.

Stress increases adrenaline, provoking more muscle tension, imbalanced hormones, and depleted calcium — exactly the conditions that promote menstrual cramps.

If your missed periods are caused by excessive exercise, low body fat, or malnutrition, simply increase your caloric intake and ease off the exercise a little.

Overweight women can also experience menstrual irregularities more often than women whose weight is normal. In those cases, a low-calorie diet, including protein from fish, soy and other legumes, spirulina, and nutritional yeast, helps regulate the menstrual cycle.

Dietary Supplements

Vitamins and minerals that may inhibit cramps include vitamins E, B6, and C and the minerals magnesium, niacin, and zinc. Spirulina and chlorella are rich in helpful nutrients. The enzyme bromelain, found in pineapple, may reduce cramping and mild uterine inflammation. These dietary supplements are widely available; follow the directions on the bottles.

Evening primrose, borage, and black currant seed oils all contain gamma-linoleic acid, or GLA, a natural medicine that is sometimes effective for cramps. It takes several months of supplementation to be effective. We also find that this oil doesn't work for every woman, and studies to determine its effectiveness have been inconclusive.

If you bruise easily and your periods are heavy, you may have weak blood vessels. They can be strengthened with vitamin C and flavonoids, found in many foods. Vitamin C also improves capillary fragility and increases iron absorption. Vitamins E, K, B12, and folic acid also can help reduce excessive bleeding. Vitamin A levels in many women with excessive bleeding have been found to be exceptionally low. In one study of 40 women, almost all found some relief from heavy periods when they took 25,000 IU of vitamin A twice a day for two weeks. This amount of vitamin A should not be taken unless under the supervision of a physician or a health-care professional, however.

Herbal Healing

Because of their ability to ease uterine pain without side effects, herbs have been valued by women for more than 2,000 years for a variety of menstrual complaints. The history of Traditional Chinese Medicine to treat menstrual disorders goes back even farther into history; there are many formulas available in many different forms. We have found in our own practices that acupuncture can be very effective in treatment for menstrual and premenstrual pain. It is also a treatment without side effects, so it may be an alternative therapy worth checking out.

Specific Remedies: Cramps

Herbs can be taken for periods that cause mild to moderate pain; they are less effective against very strong cramps. Start taking the herbs a week before menstruation and continue through the end of the flow.

Prostaglandin regulators. Ginger, cinnamon, cloves, thyme, onions, and garlic are easy to add to foods and help lower prostaglandins. Ginger can also be chopped, simmered, and used in a poultice or hot pack placed on the abdomen.

Pain relievers. The pain-relieving herbs lower prostaglandins. They are anti-inflammatory and anti-spasmodic. These herbs include willow, meadowsweet, and feverfew.

Muscle relaxants. The best-known of these herbs are cramp bark and black haw, two safe, time-proven remedies that work to relax uterine muscle. We like to use a blend of cramp bark with valerian or kava kava to increase its effect. Other effective, but lesser-known muscle relaxants include wild yam, false unicorn root, peony, scullcap, skunk cabbage, California poppy, and catnip.

Valerian is also effective when cramps are accompanied by nervousness, tension, or sleeplessness. Add it to chamomile, hops, or passion flower to help relax the entire body.

Cramp-Relieving Tea

1 teaspoon cramp bark
1/2 teaspoon motherwort
1/2 teaspoon chamomile
1/2 teaspoon wild yam root
1/2 teaspoon California poppy, whole plant or root (optional)
1/2 teaspoon valerian root
1/2 teaspoon skullcap
Licorice or stevia to taste
4 cups water

Combine herbs and water in pan. Bring to a boil, then lower heat and simmer 5 minutes. Remove from heat, cover, and steep 20 minutes. Strain out and discard herbs. Drink at least 1 cup as often as needed.

Tinctures of the above herbs can also be blended in the same proportions. Take 1 teaspoon of the blended tincture 4 or 5 times a day, beginning a few days before you expect cramps to begin and continuing until symptoms cease.

Aromatherapy for Cramps

Relaxing aromatherapy blends can help ease cramps. Essential oils of chamomile, lavender, and marjoram reduce cramping and relax the mind; they're excellent when used during massage or a bath. Clary sage uplifts the spirit, and ginger reduces cramps. These herbs or essential oils can be made into a compress or poultice.

Menstrual Cramp Oil

This recipe can be made quickly if you purchase a ready-made oil infused with St. John's wort.

1/4 cup of St. John's wort infused oil
8 drops lavender essential oil
8 drops marjoram essential oil
8 drops chamomile essential oil

Combine ingredients. Apply to lower abdomen as needed. Use also for lower back or shoulder pain and muscle cramps.

Specific Remedies: Heavy Periods

Shepherd's purse is very effective for symptomatic relief of heavy menstrual bleeding. Take 1/2 to 1 teaspoon of the tincture in a little water every fifteen minutes until the bleeding slows. If you experience heart palpitations, skip two or three doses. Consult with your health-care provider before taking large doses of shepherd's purse, but it is safe in small doses.

Other herbs that help to decrease heavy periods are yarrow, cayenne, agrimony, and lady's mantle. Herbalists believe yarrow directs blood away from the pelvic area. Raspberry leaf and nettles also decrease menstrual bleeding and tone the uterine muscle at the same time.

Additional herbs that slow bleeding, possibly through hormonal influence, are vervain, vitex, birth root, and blue cohosh. A natural iron supplement that also includes blood-building herbs, taken as advised by your health-care practitioner, can be helpful.

Aromatherapy for Heavy Periods

One of the most effective essential oils for reducing menstrual flow is sage. Like all essential oils, it must be diluted in other oils for safe use.

Tincture for Heavy Periods

1 teaspoon shepherd's purse tincture
1 teaspoon yarrow tincture
1/2 teaspoon red raspberry leaf tincture
1/2 teaspoon vitex tincture

Combine ingredients. Take 3 droppersful every 15 to 30 minutes for very heavy bleeding, or 2 droppersful every hour for moderately heavy bleeding. (Try to purchase shepherd's purse tincture made from the fresh herb; when dried, it loses some of its strength.)

Sage Massage Oil for Heavy Periods

2 ounces vegetable or almond oil
12 drops sage essential oil

Combine ingredients. Massage over lower belly a few times a day to reduce menstrual bleeding. Do not use sage essential oil if you have epilepsy or are prone to seizures.

Caution: Do not use sage essential oil if you have epilepsy or are prone to seizure.

Specific Remedies: Irregular, Scanty, or Absent Periods

Three groups of herbs can help to bring on menstruation: blood-movers and blood-builders that help to boost the blood, circulatory system, and overall metabolism; hormone regulators that smooth out imbalances in these chemicals; and emmenagogues, which can jump-start delayed periods.

Blood movers and blood builders. Herbs that are thought to help "move the blood" are not only useful for relieving pain but can help regulate menstrual periods. Some of our favorites include motherwort, black cohosh, blue cohosh, yarrow, dong quai, and prickly ash bark.

Dong quai along with a hormone regulator such as vitex also may be helpful to women trying to regain their natural menstrual cycles. We know several women who discontinued birth-control pills in anticipation of pregnancy, but months later saw no evidence of resumed ovulation. Dong quai and vitex helped stimulate their natural normal cycles, bringing about much-wanted babies.

If you consult a practitioner trained in Traditional Chinese Medicine, he or she may look for fatigue, spots before the eyes, and paleness of the tongue, cheeks, and nail beds, signs of "blood deficiency." The most important herbs for building blood include Chinese herbs dong quai, rehmannia, and *fo-ti*, and the Western herbs yellow dock and nettles.

Hormone regulators. When a woman has fully developed sex characteristics but scanty or absent menstrual flow, a hormonal problem may be the cause. The hormone-regulating herb vitex may resolve the

Build-the-Blood Tea

1/2 cup dong quai
1/2 cup fo-ti
1/4 cup yellow dock root, cut and sifted
1/2 cup nettle leaf
4 cups water

Simmer the herbs in water for 30 minutes. Cool; strain out herbs and discard. Store tea in the refrigerator for up to 3 days. Drink 1 warm cup of tea 2 or 3 times daily for three months.

condition. This herb acts on the pituitary gland to normalize and regulate ovarian hormone production. In clinical trials, vitex has shown a strong rate of success in restoring menstrual cycles when taken for three months or longer. Most importantly, vitex treatment has only a few mild side effects such as occasional skin rash and reduced libido. Women discontinuing birth-control pills may find that it takes their bodies some time to resume ovulating; two droppersful of vitex every morning may help speed this process.

Black cohosh, discussed above as a blood mover, also helps balance the menstrual cycle. Meanwhile, the phytoestrogens contained in soy, other beans, and herbs can also help regulate periods. Red clover flower is a convenient herbal way to get your phytoestrogen.

Emmenagogues. Ginger or rosemary teas also encourage menstruation. We have found that several cups of fairly strong rosemary tea are effective at bringing on a period that has been delayed. Other time-proven emmenagogues include feverfew, black cohosh, partridge berry, and tea of mugwort or a weak tea of pennyroyal.

Caution: Under *NO* circumstances should essential oil or tincture of pennyroyal be taken internally. Even small amounts have caused death.

Easy-Flow Formula

This blend of tinctures is designed to help promote regular and painless menstrual periods.

1 ounce vitex tincture
1 ounce black cohosh tincture
1 ounce red clover tincture
1/2 ounce yarrow tincture
1/4 ounce licorice tincture

Blend the tinctures together; take 1 teaspoon 2 or 3 times daily depending on the severity of symptoms. Discontinue the week before ovulation.

To prepare a tea of these herbs in the same proportions, simmer the herbs in one quart water for 30 minutes. Let cool; strain herbs out and discard. Store the tea in the refrigerator for up to three days. Drink 2 or 3 cups daily.

CHAPTER 6

PMS

*Our culture is full of references to women's "raging hormones"
and "menstrual moodiness." But PMS is much more complex —
and more treatable — than these words imply.*

Premenstrual syndrome — PMS for short — can be seen as a complicated interplay between a woman's hormones, diet, stress factors, and physical and mental health. This unique set of symptoms, ranging from mere discomfort and fatigue to debilitating cramps and depression, announces its arrival three to seven days before menstruation. A typical woman has 400 to 500 menstrual periods, so PMS can certainly affect her quality of life.

Today, women are gaining a greater understanding of their bodies. Through the use of dietary changes, herbal treatments, and healthier living, most can ultimately lead a life free of the distress and uncomfortable symptoms of PMS. In this chapter, we'll look at exactly what PMS is and what scientists know about it. We'll examine treatment options so you can make informed decisions.

Of all the hormonally related disorders that women experience, PMS is the most common. Beginning in 1931, PMS was called premenstrual tension, or PMT, but researchers later decided that "tension" does not sum up all of the problems associated with PMS. And the syndrome itself was all but ignored by the medical profession until the 1950s, when an English physician, Dr. Katerina Dalton, began to study, write, and lecture about it widely, helping to make PMS a household word. Yet, some doctors continued to scoff at the idea that women experience physical and emotional changes just before menstruation, but any woman who has had PMS can tell you how real it is.

PMS is a syndrome — a collection of several different symptoms — and the list of its effects is a long

Vitex

one; one source lists 150. These symptoms run the gamut of physical, emotional, and psychological sensations. Based on the extensive research that has been done on PMS and our own clinical experiences, we've concluded that the syndrome is influenced by many factors, making it a particular challenge for practitioners of modern medicine.

COMMON PHYSICAL SYMPTOMS OF PMS

Vague aches and pains

Mild to debilitating pelvic cramps

Breast pain and tenderness

Bloating

Insomnia

Fatigue

Hot flashes

Increased appetite, especially for carbohydrates and sweets

Clumsiness

Muscle pain

Headaches

Skin eruptions such as acne

Constipation

Nausea

COMMON PSYCHOLOGICAL SYMPTOMS OF PMS

Tension

Lethargy

Depression

Hostility

Irritability

Many of the symptoms of PMS are intertwined—they affect and exacerbate each other. When blood-sugar levels dip, the result often is fatigue, dizziness, food cravings, headache, fainting, mood swings, and sometimes heart palpitations. One of those food cravings can be for salt, leading to bloating and temporary weight gain. Although PMS sufferers may gain only a few pounds, the sudden pressure and swelling can make it feel like much more—which can add to emotional distress. To make matters worse, immune response also drops just before menstruation, possibly causing more susceptibility to colds, flu, allergies, outbreaks of herpes, and flare-ups of rheumatoid arthritis. PMS sufferers can feel as if their entire bodies are conspiring against them.

Gynecological texts estimate that PMS affects about half of women in their reproductive years, although some figures push this to 90 percent. Perhaps a third of all women have symptoms severe enough to send them to their physicians. Fewer than 5 percent of the women who suffer from PMS have debilitating psychological symptoms; this condition is called premenstrual dysphoric disorder (PMDD).

Each woman's relationship to her symptoms is unique; it is in understanding this relationship that the potential for healing lies. Naturally, women with PMS symptoms want relief for those symptoms first. But a deeper, more complex issue is how they can feel well, happy, and fulfill their creative promise as individuals on any day of the month. A return to real health—not just the alleviation of symptoms—should be the goal of PMS treatment.

BODY CHEMISTRY AND HORMONES

The mood swings, irritability, and possibly most other symptoms associated with PMS are related to strong fluctuations in several hormones. When they dip sharply, the brain and nervous system experience a withdrawal that can deeply affect mental and emotional states, much like withdrawal from addictive drugs.

One week after ovulation, and thus one week before the start of menstruation, the level of progesterone in the body reaches its cyclical high as estrogen levels are decreasing. But just before menstruation, levels of both hormones drop abruptly. This decline can be compounded by changes in levels of the minerals calcium and magnesium. All four of these substances—the two hormones and the minerals—normally fend off pain, insomnia, stress reactions, and muscle cramping.

A number of studies suggest that during the first three weeks of the menstrual cycle, increasing levels of estrogen stimulate production of the "feel-good" hormone called (beta)-endorphin, which reduces pain and elevates mood. Rising levels of progesterone at the same time make this natural opium-like substance even more potent—that is, until both estrogen and progesterone decline prior to menstruation. Then this endorphin drops, too. The result can be feelings of anxiety, along with fatigue, insomnia, and irritability. One study found that simply disrupting the ratio of estrogen to progesterone is enough to lower endorphin activity in the brain.

Prostaglandins are hormone-like fatty acids that can aggravate insomnia, stress, and pain. These substances regulate inflammation and muscle contractions in localized areas and rise before or during the menstrual flow. As a result, they can be responsible for symptoms such as abdominal cramps, general achiness,

---

CHECKLIST FOR PREMENSTRUAL DYSPHORIC DISORDER (PMDD)

The American Psychiatric Association has defined PMDD as a possible psychiatric condition. Its symptoms occur during the two weeks prior to menses and cease shortly after menstrual flow begins and are so severe as to interfere with daily life. Some typical premenstrual syndrome symptoms (see previous page), particularly psychological symptoms, are present but intense and severe. In addition, the following conditions are present.

Symptoms that occur in most cycles

Strong mood swings

Anger and irritability that lead to conflicts with others

Decreased interest in usual activities

Poor concentration

Food cravings, overeating

Sleeping too much or too little

Symptoms that do not arise from other psychiatric disorders

Disturbances that interfere with work, relationships

Self-assessed symptoms for two or more cycles

joint pain, headaches, and backache. In fact, women with dysmenorrhea (painful menstruation) have been shown to have increased prostaglandins in their menstrual blood. Drugs to block prosta-glandins—usually aspirin and ibuprofen—can successfully reduce the painful cramps that can occur before and during menstruation. Prostaglandins also are suspected of playing a role in causing breast swelling and tenderness, as well as water retention and changes in appetite.

Other hormones and hormone-like substances are associated with PMS. Scientists believe prolactin and aldosterone may be involved because of their known role in water retention. Studies confirm that PMS sufferers often have higher than normal levels of prolactin. One of the hormones that helps nursing women produce breast milk, prolactin is also associated with anxiety, irritability, mood swings, water reten-tion, and weight gain. It is especially notorious for promoting breast tenderness and breast cysts. A drug that inhibits production of pro-lactin, bromocriptine, reduces some PMS symptoms, especially breast tenderness, bloating, and depression. A drug that inhibits aldosterone,

PROGESTERONE THERAPY AND PMS

An old but still popular theory is that PMS is caused by a drop in progesterone before the period — or a disruption in the ratio between estrogen and progesterone. But the con-nection between progesterone and PMS is still not completely clear. Some studies show that progesterone supplementation reduces PMS symptoms; in others, no effect was found. Dr. Katerina Dalton, British pioneer of progesterone therapy, found in both her practice and research that most women with PMS had very low levels of progesterone. In one of her studies, PMS symptoms in all forty-five women either disappeared or were at least partially relieved with injections of progesterone.

Some research also links higher-than-normal levels of progesterone with increased symptoms of PMS. Dalton also found that the few women who have low estrogen with high progesterone are most likely to experience severe depression, confusion, insomnia, and suicidal feelings during PMS.

The results of the various studies are confusing even to researchers. One research group conducted a double-blind, placebo-controlled trial with 25 volunteers with PMS and 17 women without symptoms. The researchers found that 200 mg of progesterone, taken twice daily by vaginal suppository, reduced tension and mood swings in the study group compared with the control group. Another study found that micronized progesterone sup-plements, taken orally 4 times daily from day 18 of the cycle through day 2 of the next cycle, had no more effect than a placebo in 444 volunteers who had PMS symptoms.

spironolactone, has been found to reduce PMS symptoms in some cases, even though PMS patients usually don't have abnormal aldosterone levels.

Finally, still other neurotransmitters are associated with emotional functioning and mood. Recent studies have shown that estrogen levels are directly related to levels of the neurotransmitter serotonin. As estrogen levels decrease before menstruation, so do serotonin levels. That's why current treatment for severe PMS and PMDD can include antidepressant drugs that boost serotonin levels.

WHAT A DOCTOR WILL DO

Most women who seek medical help for PMS have already had mild to moderate symptoms for one to three years; they visit their practitioner only when the symptoms increase in intensity. This is especially true if they suffer from emotional symptoms such as irritability and depression.

Although there is no exact method of diagnosing PMS, most doctors rely on extensive questioning. Before prescribing a medication, a physician or psychiatrist usually makes a diagnosis based in part on a daily journal of symptoms kept by the patient for at least two cycles. Gathering this information may seem cumbersome and can delay treatment, but current medical thought indicates that about half the women who come in for PMS-like symptoms actually have another disorder, since their symptoms do not fluctuate with their menstrual cycle or worsen just before menses.

If you are suffering from PMS, you'll need to keep track of your symptoms for three to four months. You should see the same symptoms repeat themselves month after month. You can start your own journal and use this information to design a course of treatment with herbs, diet, supplements, and habit changes.

Researchers have identified four separate types of PMS based on symptoms and hormonal and nutritional status. The chart on page 77 summarizes these categories and some herbal and dietary remedies for each. Don't worry if your symptoms don't fit neatly into one of these categories—many women's symptoms overlap them. But if you do exhibit a strong tendency toward one group of symptoms, the chart can help you choose the most appropriate dietary supplements and herbs.

Conventional Treatments

When a diagnosis of PMS is made, treatment can vary depending on the main complaint. Common treatments include diuretics, prostaglandin inhibitors, progesterone or estrogen/progesterone birth control pills, or antidepressants. However, we always support the use of natural remedies and building healthy habits as a first line of defense against disease and unpleasant symptoms. In our opinion, powerful hormones should not be used indiscriminately. The effects of their long-term use are not known.

As for PMDD, the favored medical treatment for severe symptoms is low dosages of antidepressants such as Prozac (fluoxetine), Zoloft (sertraline), Xanax (alprazolam), and BuSpar (buspirone). About half the women who take them experience some improvement. As might be expected, these drugs are particularly effective when a woman has severe emotional changes during PMS. However, these drugs are difficult to discontinue. Ironically, they can also produce side effects that mimic PMS symptoms, such as fatigue, insomnia, dizziness, and headaches. Many antidepressants reduce interest in sex and can make it difficult to achieve orgasm. Anxiety and other emotional problems are sometimes treated with sedatives and tranquilizers such as Valium (diazepam), but these drugs are addictive.

It has long been popular to treat water retention and swollen breasts with diuretics, but today many doctors believe they may do more harm than good. Still, women commonly use them in an effort to lose extra PMS pounds. In some cases, prolactin inhibitors such as Parlodel (bromocriptine mesylate) are used to reduce breast swelling and pain, headaches, and mood swings, but side effects are common.

Nonsteroidal anti-inflammatory drugs (NSAIDs), such as aspirin, acetaminophen (Tylenol) and ibuprofen, as well as prostaglandin inhibitors such as mefanamic acid, have long been prescribed to reduce swollen breasts and to ease headaches and joint pain. They have no effect on emotions or behavior, but large doses can be toxic to the liver.

Doctors have been slow to adopt progesterone alone as a PMS therapy, especially since several well-controlled studies have failed to demonstrate its benefit. In our experience, some women report nearly miraculous results from progesterone, but others experience no effect.

NATURAL HEALING

Healthy Habits

Various studies show that relaxation methods such as aerobic exercise, yoga, and meditation can relieve PMS symptoms. The assumption is that they do so by altering brain chemistry and probably boosting endorphins, the body's natural mood-elevating and pain-relieving

CATEGORIES OF PMS

Researchers have identified four types of PMS, based on patients' hormone levels and nutrition levels. The dietary and herbal treatments summarized here are discussed in more detail later in this chapter.

PMS-A (Anxiety): Irritability, nervous tension, mood swings, insomnia

Possible causes: Related to high estrogen levels and low progesterone levels

Alternative treatments: Supplement with vitamin B6, 100–200 mg, or vitex to increase progesterone and balance estrogen. Black cohosh, as well as soybean food products, can help balance estrogen levels.

PMS-B (also called PMS-H for hyperhydration): Water and salt retention, bloating, weight gain, breast swelling, and tenderness

Possible causes: Liver weakness, hormone imbalance, potassium imbalance

Alternative treatments: Reduce salt intake. Supplement with vitamins B6 and E. Avoid caffeine and cigarettes. Try herbal aquaretics such as dandelion leaf.

PMS-C (Craving): Sweet cravings, increased appetite, low blood sugar, fatigue, dizziness, headaches, sometimes heart palpitations

Possible causes: Magnesium deficiency, poor carbohydrate metabolism, weak digestion

Alternative treatments: Supplement with magnesium, starting with about 400 mg per day. Eliminate simple sugars of all forms. Eat more complex carbohydrates before period, more protein after flow stops. Before meals, use a digestive tonic such as a bitters preparation. Reduce salt intake.

PMS-D (Depression): Depression, withdrawal, confusion, forgetfulness

Possible causes: Increased progesterone during mid-luteal phase; decreased serotonin levels

Alternative treatments: Eat more foods that contain tryptophan (turkey, spirulina, almonds or almond milk, nutritional yeast). Supplement with St. John's wort. Use a liver-balancing and relaxing herbal supplement daily for the two weeks after menstruation ends.

Source: Abraham, 1983

DRUGS COMMONLY PRESCRIBED FOR PMS

Drug and drug type	Action	Possible side effects	Herbal alternatives
Danazol (testosterone derivative)	Suppresses some mid-cycle hormones; relieves breast tenderness; not as effective for non-physical symptoms	Weight gain, edema, acne, oily skin, decreased breast size, increased hair growth, hot flashes, sweating, vaginitis, potential suppression of menses	Vitex
Prozac, Zoloft, Paxil (selective serotonin reuptake inhibitors, or SSRIs)	Slows the uptake and breakdown of the neurotransmitter serotonin by nerve cells	Headache, nausea, insomnia, nervousness	St. John's wort
BuSpar (Buspirone, nonsedative antianxiety drug)	Eases worry, apprehension, inability to cope, difficulty in concentration	Headache, dizziness, nausea (3–12% of patients); disinhibition, ataxia, agitation, anxiety, confusion, gastrointestinal distress	California poppy, valerian, other calmatives
Xanax, Valium, Ativan (benzodiazepines)	Sedatives; reduce anxiety and promote sleep	Headache, nausea, tinnitus, insomnia, nervousness, anxiety, memory loss, drowsiness; extremely addictive	California poppy, valerian, other calmatives
Parlodel (bromocriptine mesylate)	Acts on pituitary gland; suppresses prolactin secretion	Common: nausea, vomiting, dizziness, decreased blood pressure, appetite loss. Rare: hypertension, seizures, stroke, psychosis	Vitex
Aspirin, acetaminophen, ibuprofen (nonsteroidal anti-inflammatories, or NSAIDS)	Reduce pain, breast tenderness; suppress prostaglandin	Can be toxic to the liver in large doses; aspirin can cause stomach and gastrointestinal bleeding	Meadowsweet, Jamaican dogwood, feverfew

substances. Regular exercise often eases the mild depression of PMS and can help with other symptoms as well. PMS sufferers generally find that aerobic exercise works better than strength training, again because the aerobic activity releases more endorphins. And any type of aerobic exercise will do, as long as it is steady and done for at least twenty minutes, three to four days weekly. One medical text suggests forty-five minutes of daily exercise that includes some aerobic exercise.

Dietary Changes

If you suffer from PMS, regulating your intake of some foods may help. Surveys show that women who suffer from PMS eat as much as 75 percent more salt than women who have no symptoms. They also consume more candy, ice cream, cake, and sugary soft drinks, indulging in a whopping 275 per cent more refined sugar than women without PMS.

If you make only one dietary change to ease your PMS symptoms, eliminate refined sugar products. This move will contribute tremendously to your overall health and well-being. Instead, turn to fresh whole fruit in season, carob, nuts, and dried fruit. Eating several small meals per day will help reduce cravings by keeping your blood-sugar levels even.

Studies show that women who suffer from PMS consume an average of 75 percent more salt and 275 percent more refined sugar than women without symptoms.

One problem with a high sugar intake is that it alters blood sugar and renders emotions less stable. Consuming refined sugar products increases the metabolic rate, creating excess heat in the body. It also acts as an immune suppressant, contributing to such symptoms as chronic yeast infection and acne. Refined-sugar consumption also increases the elimination of magnesium and depletes B-vitamins—the very nutrients that help one cope with stress.

While you're at it, avoid chocolate and coffee—at least for the week or two before menstruation. We know that this may not be easy, but coffee and chocolate appear to worsen PMS symptoms. Just one cup of coffee can increase their likelihood by 30 percent, according to one study. Caffeine also increases nervous tension, heart rate, insomnia, and headache and can contribute to breast pain.

We believe that women who suffer from PMS also dine on more refined carbohydrates and dairy products than women who don't. The problem is, women with PMS also are more likely to crave these foods while they are having symptoms.

MIT researchers suggest these women go ahead and give in to their cravings. Dining on complex, unrefined carbohydrates, such as whole grains, can help to relieve depression, anger, anxiety, insomnia, and mood swings related to PMS. This is probably because carbohydrates help speed up the conversion of amino acids such as tryptophan into serotonin. Remember that serotonin levels drop dramatically after ovulation and just before the start of menses. Increased carbohydrates may help counteract this drop, easing moodiness and encouraging emotional well-being and sound sleep.

We find that women with PMS do well to eat more complex carbohydrates during the days after ovulation through the end of the menstrual flow, and fewer carbohydrates and more protein from the end of the period through ovulation. The increased protein helps boost stores of important amino acids that seem to be used up more quickly during the rest of the cycle. Don't go overboard in trimming protein before your period; your body still requires at least thirty to forty grams a day. Try increasing protein and reducing carbohydrates by 20 to 25 percent after your period, then returning to your usual levels of these foods.

Still other foods to avoid are red meat, dairy products, and eggs. They can interfere with magnesium absorption and worsen PMS. Eating too much fat also causes problems. In one study, thirty women ate a diet with 40 percent of calories from fat for four complete menstrual cycles. They then switched to a diet with half that amount of fat for another four cycles. The result: as expected, the women gained weight during the first four cycles — but bloating and breast tenderness also increased.

HELP FOR PMS MIGRAINES

If migraine headaches are on your list of PMS symptoms, follow the National Headache Foundation's advice to avoid these foods known to trigger them.

Ripened cheese (cheddar, Gruyère, Brie, and Camembert)

Sausage

Onions

Pickles

Cured meats

Avocados

Fresh bread

Red wine

Sour cream

Nuts

Chocolate

Coffee

Tea

Cola

Alcohol

Dietary Supplements

Here is a review of other nutritional supplements that have been studied for their ability to ease symptoms of PMS.

Magnesium. Studies have shown that magnesium levels in women with PMS are often lower than normal throughout the cycle, especially before the menstrual flow begins. The premenstrual dip in magnesium, sometimes combined with the increase in aldosterone, causes sodium and fluid retention. This disrupts the sodium/potassium balance. As a result, even less magnesium and vitamin B6 are assimilated. Magnesium has other important functions for PMS. This mineral, with help from the B vitamins, keeps blood sugar stabilized and prevents food cravings by supporting the liver's conversion of carbohydrates and glucose into sugar. (One theory why some premenstrual women are so attracted to chocolate is that it contains magnesium.)

Calcium. Too much calcium, especially for women who have PMS-A, can actually aggravate symptoms by reducing the absorption of magnesium. Supplements containing twice as much magnesium as calcium may be the best choice for women with PMS-A symptoms. For other women, calcium may decrease muscle cramps.

B6 or a B-vitamin complex with B6. Deficiencies in this nutrient can lead to decreases in serotonin levels, resulting in depression and irritability. Vitamin B6 can also suppress aldosterone, helping to ease bloating.

One doctor and his co-workers at a gynecology clinic found that vitamin B6 (50 mg daily) alone decreased the symptoms in the majority of patients who had moderate to severe PMS, including premenstrual acne. No one had to tell these women when they were receiving placebos instead of the vitamin, because, to their disappointment, their symptoms soon returned.

In other studies, vitamin B6 had no effect or minimal effects on PMS. We believe that this contradiction in the research is probably due to differences among individual women. Some PMS sufferers may be deficient in vitamin B6, and some may not. Since it is often difficult to diagnose a deficiency of vitamin B6, we still feel that this nutrient, or better still, a well-balanced B-complex, may be helpful in reducing symptoms of PMS. We suggest starting with 100 mg per day. Some women experience side effects such as indigestion and gastritis with larger doses.

Vitamin D. One recent report of women with migraine headaches associated with PMS shows help from supplements of vitamin D in conjunction with calcium. Calcium was given in the amount of 1200 mg per day, along with 1200 to 1600 IU of vitamin D3 (cholecalciferol). The migraine attacks were significantly improved after two months.

Vitamin E. One 1983 double-blind study found that vitamin E supplementation improved symptoms of PMS-A, PMS-C, and PMS-D after two months. The effective dose was between 150 IU and 300 IU, twice daily. Vitamins B6 and E team up with magnesium to lower prolactin, as well as weight gain, nervous anxiety, and nausea. In several studies in which PMS sufferers took vitamin E for two or three months, their depression, irritability, bloating, and sweet cravings all decreased.

Herbal Healing

We have seen herbal remedies do wonders for many sufferers of PMS over the years. But it is often necessary to experiment with several herbs, as well as dietary changes, before finding the right combination. We wrote this book to present a number of tried-and-true choices, and to help you create the most effective personal program.

The following herbal remedies for PMS are arranged by the type of action the herbs have on the body.

Hormone Regulators

Vitex. Extracts from the small, hard, dry spicy fruits of a Mediterranean shrub, *Vitex agnus-castus*, also known chaste tree, help relieve PMS symptoms, probably by rebalancing hormones. Vitex is especially useful for treating fluid retention, mood swings, and food cravings. One study done in Germany has shown that a vitex preparation known as Strotan corrects prolactin over-secretion in women. Vitex also decreases bouts of premenstrual acne, constipation, and herpes. Consider trying a progesterone-stimulating herb such as vitex before turning to pharmaceutical-grade progesterone creams or capsules. To take vitex in a tincture, start with a dose of two to three droppersful, morning and evening, in a little water, away from mealtimes. If you choose the powdered herb in capsules, take three capsules twice daily.

Black cohosh. This common women's herb is often blended in formulas with vitex for both PMS and menopause. Although generally considered an estrogen-regulating herb, it also prevents estrogen from over-stimulating sensitive tissue in the uterus, thus helping to relieve pain and swelling. It also acts as an anti-inflammatory and antispasmodic, reducing swelling, spasms, and pain. Take about three to four droppersful of the tincture morning and evening. A drawback of this herb is its tendency to stimulate heavy menstrual bleeding in some women.

GLA and evening primrose oil. One of the most popular herbal supplements to ease symptoms of PMS is GLA (gamma-linoleic acid), a fatty acid derived from evening primrose, black currant, or borage seeds. It is widely sold in natural products stores, drug stores, and even grocery stores. It is available only in capsules because the product is highly concentrated and not enough can be obtained from making a tea or eating the ground seeds. Unfortunately, this makes it a little more expensive than most herbal remedies.

Not all studies on the use of GLA for premenstrual symptoms have been positive. Although seven placebo-controlled clinical trials with human volunteers have been performed over the last few years, one group of researchers concluded that the studies were not up to modern scientific standards. Some of the studies included only a few women, and in a number of them, the evening primrose oil worked only slightly better than the placebo. Although our experience tells us that this natural product is helpful, you may wish to try flax seed meal or oil first; use a half tablespoon to one tablespoon per day. It's just as effective for some women and costs a lot less.

No matter how you take GLA, be aware that it may take three or four months before effects are felt. For some women, relief may take even longer.

Antidepressants

Kava kava and St. John's wort. This dynamic duo of antianxiety and mood-elevating herbs encourages relaxation and a good night's sleep. Take four droppersful of a tincture in the morning and three in the evening. A standardized tablet or capsule will also often work. Remember that St. John's wort seems to act similarly to serotonin-affecting antidepressants and therefore requires several weeks of use before any effect can be expected. Kava kava, on the other hand, can produce short-term mood-elevating effects almost instantly. It can also be used in liquid form, three to four droppersful at a time, two to three times daily, but again, capsules or tablets are sometimes effective, depending on quality.

Herbs that boost energy levels and increase endurance can help counter the effects of premenstrual drops in blood sugar.

Metabolic Regulators

Herbs that boost energy levels and increase endurance can help counter the effects of premenstrual drops in blood sugar.

Chinese ginseng and Siberian ginseng. Both herbs help stabilize blood sugar, alleviate depression, and support adrenal function to counteract the impact of stress. Ginseng is often used in Traditional Chinese Medicine to warm and strengthen digestion and encourage assimilation of nutrients.

Stevia. Instead of sugar, use stevia to sweeten your tea and even your food. Although this herb is actually sweeter than table sugar, the bittersweet taste may take some getting used to. If you find it unpleasant, try mixing it with honey. Traditionally used in its native Paraguay to stabilize blood sugar, stevia is available in natural food stores as both a dried herb and as a liquid.

Circulatory Herbs

Blood-movers reduce water retention and relieve congestion, swelling, and pain in the veins and capillaries of the uterus.

Ginkgo. Although best known for its action on the brain and circulation, this herb can be used to treat some PMS symptoms, specifically breast tenderness. Other well-known blood-movers include dong quai, Chinese red sage, ginger, and prickly ash bark.

Ginkgo

Anti-inflammatories

These herbs can help when PMS causes pain and swelling in internal organs and vessels. Some inhibit the manufacture of prostaglandins.

Feverfew. Some women report that this herb, which relieves migraine headaches and other types of chronic inflammation, also diminishes their PMS symptoms. The London Migraine Clinic found that the freeze-dried leaves, taken for three months, not only reduce headaches but increase a sense of well-being. Perhaps Renaissance herbalist John Gerard was on to something when he wrote that feverfew was a good remedy for "them that are giddie in the head . . . melancholilike, sad, pensive." He also said of feverfew, "It is a great remedie against the diseases of the matrix [the uterus]."

Other respected anti-inflammatories include chamomile, echinacea, and yarrow.

Nervines (Calmatives)

If nervousness, anxiety, and sleeping problems result from PMS, try herbal calmatives to relax the central nervous system.

California poppy. This effective calmative works well as a tincture or as a powdered extract in capsules or tablets. It can help calm mild anxiety, promote a feeling of relaxation, and lead to good, refreshing sleep.

Hops. This relaxing herb is especially useful for promoting sleep and calming heart palpitations. It is also mildly estrogenic, which makes it useful for women who have low estrogen levels. Women who have had breast cancers that are estrogen-driven may wish to avoid its use, though like all phytoestrogens, its mild activity is probably more balancing than stimulating to the estrogen tissues.

Our other favorite calmatives are valerian, linden, passion flower, and chamomile.

Liver Regulators

In our experience, an effective herbal program to relieve symptoms of PMS should contain liver-supporting herbs. The liver plays a key role in regulating hormones.

In Traditional Chinese Medicine, the liver is thought to regulate the blood. For this reason, irregular menses, heavy bleeding, absence of menses, and other bleeding irregularities are often associated with a liver that is bound up and congested; this is called "stagnant liver Qi." It is also the liver's job to regulate levels of estrogen and other sexual hormones by selectively breaking them down to less active compounds. To help the liver work smoothly, herbalists often recommend regulatory herbs that enhance the liver's production of important enzymes and increase bile flow. Bile is the source of compounds that the body uses to create estrogen, progesterone, and other steroid hormones.

Bile-movers include artichoke leaf, wormwood, dandelion root, and the great liver-protective herb, milk thistle. Herbs that can enhance liver-enzyme production and regulate liver function are burdock, fringe-tree bark, the popular Chinese herb bupleurum, and the South American herb boldo. One of the most popular ready-made Chinese formulas is *Xiao Yao Wan*, "Free and Easy Wanderer", which is often prescribed by Chinese practitioners to help relieve symptoms of PMS. It is available from acupuncturists, Chinese herbal shops, and natural products stores.

Diuretics (Aquaretics)

We have found that gentle herbal diuretics help the body release extra water weight that collects during PMS. In Europe, these herbs are called aquaretics to distinguish them from strong pharmaceutical diuretics, which increase urine flow but simultaneously flush out important nutrients such as magnesium, calcium, and potassium. Aquaretics include parsley root, parsley leaves, cleavers, asparagus, artichoke, nettles, and dandelion leaf.

Dandelion leaves

Digestive Regulators

Bitter herbs such as gentian, wormwood, artichoke leaf, and centaury improve digestion and assimilation several different ways. They activate intestinal movement, regulate appetite, and enhance production of important digestive enzymes such as hydrochloric acid and bile. These bitter herbs are often combined with spicy herbs such as ginger and cardamon, and harmonizing herbs such as orange peel.

Another category of digestive herbs includes those that warm up the internal fires to help the digestion and assimilation of food and relieve pain, water retention, and fatigue. Ginger tea is one of the most proven and respected herbs for relieving nausea and abdominal discomfort from PMS. In fact, one of our favorite combinations is 75 percent ginger and 25 percent ginseng. Use it as a tea, tincture, or powdered extract. Other warming spicy herbs for digestion include cardamon, cinnamon, and black pepper as found in the Indian drink, chai.

PMS Tea

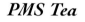

1 teaspoon vitex berry
1 teaspoon wild yam root
1/2 teaspoon burdock root
1/2 teaspoon dandelion root
1/2 teaspoon feverfew leaf
4 cups water

Combine herbs and water. Bring to a boil, then turn off heat and let steep at least 20 minutes. Strain out herbs. Drink as needed, at least 2 cups daily. We recommend adding flavoring and sweetening herbs to make the blend more enjoyable. Try orange peel, licorice root, or stevia.

This formula also can be taken as a tincture (3 droppersful, twice daily). To make your own tincture, buy individual tinctures and blend them in the same proportions, or purchase one of the many similar formulas already blended to treat menstrual pain.

PMS Tonic Tincture

1 teaspoon tincture of ginger
1/2 teaspoon tincture of cardamon
1/2 teaspoon tincture of cinnamon
3/4 teaspoon tincture of orange peel
1/4 teaspoon tincture of licorice root
2 teaspoons tincture of artichoke leaf
1 teaspoon tincture of gentian root

Blend the herbal tinctures. Take 1 teaspoon in a little water before the two major meals of the day.

Period-Regulating Extract

This formula helps regulate the hormones, relax the liver, and lift the mood.

1 plus 1/4 teaspoon vitex tincture
3/4 teaspoon black cohosh tincture
1/2 teaspoon motherwort tincture
1 teaspoon boldo or burdock root tincture
1 teaspoon St. John's wort tincture
1/2 teaspoon California poppy tincture
tincture of stevia or licorice root to sweeten, if desired

Blend the individual tinctures together. Take 1 teaspoon of the blend, morning and evening, at least 30 minutes away from meals. Keep taking the blend for at least 4 months.

Variations: For addressing other symptoms, try adding a teaspoon of one or more of the following tinctures to the above recipe.

Uterine cramps: Valerian, cramp bark, or more California poppy.

Pain: Jamaican dogwood, meadowsweet, or the Chinese herb corydalis

Water retention: Tincture of dandelion leaf

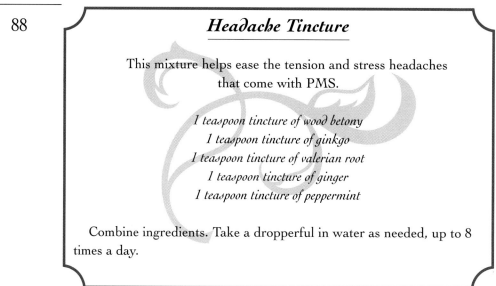

Headache Tincture

This mixture helps ease the tension and stress headaches
that come with PMS.

1 teaspoon tincture of wood betony
1 teaspoon tincture of ginkgo
1 teaspoon tincture of valerian root
1 teaspoon tincture of ginger
1 teaspoon tincture of peppermint

Combine ingredients. Take a dropperful in water as needed, up to 8
times a day.

Aromatherapy

Aromatherapy treatments are most effective with PMS if you begin
them at the first PMS signs. Try a relaxing aromatherapy bath or massage with essential oils that calm both mind and body. Good ones include
clary sage, lavender, rose, rose geranium, neroli (orange blossom), ylang
ylang, chamomile, and petitgrain. All these scents are used as antidepressants. Add about four drops total essential oil to your bath water, or follow the recipe below for making a massage oil.

For problems with food cravings or water retention, use grapefruit
and juniper oils in the bath. To relieve a headache, try inhaling lavender,
marjoram, or lemon balm. Or apply an aromatherapy compress to the
forehead and/or the back of the neck. Just add four drops essential oil
of lavender or chamomile to two cups warm water and dunk a soft cloth
in the mixture.

Premenstrual Massage Oil

1/2 cup vegetable oil
1/4 teaspoon lavender essential oil
8 drops clary sage essential oil

Combine ingredients. Use for a relaxing massage.

CHAPTER 7

ENDOMETRIOSIS

Difficult to diagnose and treat medically, endometriosis often responds to lifestyle changes and natural remedies.

What is endometriosis? This condition's name comes from endometrium, the special tissue that lines the uterus and expands and becomes blood-filled in order to receive and nourish a fertilized egg cell when a woman becomes pregnant. If no egg cell is implanted, the hormones estrogen and progesterone decrease, causing this special tissue to degenerate; its upper layer is shed each month during the menstrual period.

In endometriosis, these cells are present outside the uterus and attach themselves to other areas, most commonly the cervix, ovaries, fallopian tubes, bladder, or intestines. In response to monthly hormonal changes, this tissue, too, swells and degenerates during the menstrual cycle.

The symptoms of endometriosis—known well to about 5 percent of American women—include severe menstrual cramps, excessive bleeding, gas, pain during ovulation or intercourse, and sometimes depression and insomnia. Some symptoms increase several days before menstruation and continue until it is over. A recent German survey found that of women ages 20 to 29 being treated for endometriosis, 90 percent reported menstrual pain, 80 percent infertility, 71 percent pelvic pain, and 46 percent menstrual irregularity.

As the misplaced uterine tissue bleeds each month, it can become a source of scarring and inflammation of nearby organs. Blood clots can occur, causing adhesions to other organs and possibly distorting them. The scar tissue may also lead to bowel inflammation and constriction of the cervix. Concurrent infection of the uterus, bladder, or vagina can occur. All of these conditions cause pelvic pain; constipation, uterine fibroids, an IUD, a cancerous growth, or even a tampon can increase it. Between 30 and 60 percent of

Yarrow

infertile women are believed to have endometriosis; only about 50 percent of women who try to get pregnant after treatment for endometriosis are successful.

The Elusive Causes

The most common theory about the cause of endometriosis involves retrograde menstruation. The term refers to blood and endometrial tissue that travel into the fallopian tubes during menstruation instead of exiting the body through the vagina. Retrograde menstruation may involve an increase in estrogen or an increased sensitivity to estrogen in some women. Yet many women with normal cycles experience retrograde menstruation without ever developing endometriosis.

So what creates endometriosis is still a mystery. Some clues point to an overabundance of estrogen. North American women who have the condition are typically between the ages of 25 and 40; most are childless. Both progesterone treatments and pregnancy alleviate its symptoms; both also result in higher progesterone and lower estrogen. Women who have not had a full-term pregnancy are more likely to have endometriosis; apparently the longer a woman does not bear a child, the more estrogen she is exposed to during her lifetime. Hormonal substances called prostaglandins, which increase inflammation and swelling, may play a role.

A disorder in the immune system may contribute to endometriosis. In fact, one study found that high levels of autoantibodies, which signal an immune response to a patient's own tissue, were detected in almost all women with endometriosis who were tested. These autoantibodies may cause an inflammatory response toward the endometrial tissue, which causes the pain.

In some rare cases, endometrial tissue can appear in sites far from the pelvic region, including the lungs and retina, giving rise to a theory that the tissue spreads through the blood and lymphatic systems. Some doctors have even speculated that the condition begins before a woman is born, when endometrial cells develop in the wrong locations.

Risk Factors

Endometriosis is on the rise in the United States. Curiously, European women rarely have it, compared to 3 to 5 percent of American

---

YOU THOUGHT YOU KNEW . . .

Endometriosis is surrounded by misunderstandings and myths. It was once considered a disease of high achievers, but it occurs in all types of women. It was once believed that pregnancy would cure endometriosis because pregnancy alters hormonal levels, but such relief is usually only temporary.

women. The few identified risk factors fall far short of predicting which women will develop endometriosis.

By definition, endometriosis occurs almost exclusively during the reproductive years. It is sometimes diagnosed in teenagers. A recent study examined women ages 22 or younger who were referred to a pediatric/adolescent gynecology practice for chronic pelvic pain. For relief, the women had tried oral contraceptives or nonsteroidal anti-inflammatories such as ibuprofen, without success. Laparoscopy tests found that nearly 70 percent had endometriosis.

Environmental toxins may also play a role. In 1994, the Environmental Protection Agency linked endometriosis and dioxin in several animal studies, including one in which female monkeys exposed to dioxin developed endometriosis. The chemical structure of dioxin, some polychlorinated biphenyls (PCBs), and some pesticides mimic human estrogen and are stored in the body's fatty tissues; they may act similarly to estrogen in stimulating some cells.

A study of nearly 4,000 women found that those who drink alcohol have a 50-percent higher risk of developing endometriosis than those who abstain.

WHAT A DOCTOR WILL DO

Endometriosis presents a variety of symptoms, making diagnosis difficult. It can imitate pelvic inflammatory disease, a growth on the ovaries, or a uterine tumor; it shares some symptoms with ectopic pregnancy and uterine fibroids. One clue is that endometriosis is aggravated during menstruation, while, except for fibroids, the other disorders are not.

A preliminary diagnosis of endometriosis can be made by a pelvic exam when two areas, called the uterosacral ligament and the cul-de-sac, are extremely tender. Magnetic resonance imaging is also used and is about 96 percent accurate. However, laparoscopy is the most reliable diagnostic method. It involves making a small incision near the navel and viewing the pelvic cavity directly with a laparoscope—a small, flexible viewing instrument. In this way, doctors can find spots of endometriosis and the damage it has done; with surgical tools or lasers attached to the scope, they can also remove endometrial and scar tissue. The procedure requires general anesthesia.

Surgical treatment of endometriosis has a fairly high success rate for relieving pain. Endometrial tissue returns after surgery but it does so slowly; a study of the long-term efficacy of laparoscopic laser surgery in

the treatment of endometriosis has found that one year after the procedure, symptom relief continues in 90 percent of the patients.

Skillfully performed laparoscopic surgery increases the chances of
pregnancy in infertile women who have moderate or severe endometriosis, but not in those with mild endometriosis. Not surprisingly, one study
found that laparoscopic surgery performed by inexperienced surgeons
results in a high rate of complications, so if you're going to have this
surgery, find an experienced doctor.

Severe endometriosis may call for more extensive surgery, but the
reproductive organs should be left intact. Although hysterectomy was
once frequently recommended to cure endometriosis, it is rarely necessary. Endometrial implants usually occur in the pelvic cavity outside the
uterus, so hysterectomy may not resolve the disease.

Drug Treatments

Generally, the goal of treating endometriosis with drugs is to keep
the disease in check by decreasing the effects of estrogen. While these
treatments can relieve pain and decrease lesions, their side effects are
typical of menopause: reduced bone mass, vaginal dryness, hot flashes,
and weight gain. When the drugs are discontinued, endometriosis
symptoms often reappear. The following drugs are commonly prescribed for endometriosis.

Danazol. A derivative of testosterone, Danazol reduces the size of
endometrial areas and decreases pelvic pain, but its numerous side
effects include weight gain, unwanted hair growth, hot flashes, vaginal
dryness, deepening of the voice, acne, fatigue, water retention, and
decreased sexual drive.

GnRH analogs. These synthesized versions of gonadotropin-releas-
ing hormone, or GnRH, are sometimes effective in relieving the pelvic
pain of endometriosis and shrinking extensive areas of abnormal tissue
before surgery. They may result in the cessation of normal periods,
along with menopause-like symptoms. Because of these side effects,
the FDA has approved them for treating endometriosis a maximum of
six months.

Progesterone. This hormone stops ovulation and controls estrogen
levels. It is sometimes administered by injection of Depo-Provera, a long-
acting contraceptive, or an oral Provera, both forms of synthetic progesterone. Sometimes these drugs stop ovulation, so they are a poor choice
for women who want children. Topical creams containing progesterone
are a promising form of therapy for endometriosis; some studies have

shown that these creams give the relief of internal progesterone therapy without the side effects.

Estrogen/progesterone. Low-dose oral contraceptives containing these hormones are often used to prevent ovulation in patients with mild endometriosis. For many physicians, this is the nonsurgical treatment of choice. While it won't cure the disease, it can stabilize it and reduce pain and cramping with fewer side effects than other drugs.

NATURAL HEALING

Endometriosis is not easily attributable to any one imbalance. We recommend seeking the help of a trained health practitioner, such as an acupuncturist or naturopath, for a complete diagnosis. We firmly believe that it is important to treat the person and not the disease. Precisely because endometriosis is slow to develop, it offers an opportunity to give natural healing methods a chance.

Special Healthy Habits

Exercise to increase circulation to the pelvic area can help tremendously, but overly strenuous workouts can lead to increased pain and cramping, especially just before or during menstruation. The best forms of exercise for endometriosis are those that combine breath control with gentle movement, such as tai chi, qi gong, yoga, and expressionistic dance.

Don't smoke, and if you do, quit. The first puff you take on your first cigarette begins to compromise your immune system. Avoid alcohol as well, especially if infertility is a problem.

TRADITIONAL CHINESE MEDICINE AND ENDOMETRIOSIS

Traditional Chinese Medicine has much to offer women who suffer from endometriosis. We've found that acupuncture treatments can be effective where other conventional treatments have failed. In one study, infertile women were treated with either acupuncture or hormonal therapy. Even though the group receiving acupuncture had more pronounced hormonal disorders, only 44 percent of the acupuncture group remained infertile after therapy, compared to 56 percent of the group treated with hormones. In each group, 35 percent of the women who failed to become pregnant were diagnosed with endometriosis.

Acupuncture may also help relieve menstrual pain from endometriosis. One study of 48 women found that after only two acupuncture treatments, half experienced pain relief.

When possible, use pads during your period. Tampons may encourage retrograde menstruation, pain, and cramps. Heat tends to relieve endometrial pain for most women; try hot baths or hot packs. Instructions for sitz baths and essential oil packs follow in the aromatherapy section.

Dietary Changes and Supplements

We recommend a low-fat diet, high in fiber and including abundant amounts of fresh vegetables and fruits and few animal fats or fatty foods. Both fats and dairy products can stimulate estrogen production.

Phytoestrogens are particularly important for treating endometriosis. These compounds, found in soy-based foods, other beans, and herbs such as red clover, can help prevent natural or synthetic estrogens from overstimulating body tissues. Aim for about 150 to 200 mg of phytoestrogens per day. If you can't get that from your food, consider drinking a daily dose of red clover tea, which also has good blood-moving and vessel-strengthening properties. Standardized extracts of red clover and soy also are available in capsules and tablets if you are not inclined to make the tea or foods daily.

Finally, eliminate as much caffeine from your diet as possible. We've seen the mere elimination of caffeine make a considerable difference in relieving symptoms of endometriosis.

SUPPLEMENTS FOR ENDOMETRIOSIS

An antioxidant program can help prevent tissue damage and reduce inflammation and scarring. Take the following daily:

Vitamin E, 400–800 IU

Vitamin C, 2–5 grams

Grape-seed or green-tea extract, 200–400 mg

Magnesium, 500 mg

Look for these additional nutrients in your supplement: beta-carotene, selenium, and zinc.

Herbal Remedies

Herbs have great potential for curing endometriosis, but they require patience because treatment can take months to show effects. Women often find that the condition does not resolve completely, but that symptoms practically disappear, helping them avoid surgery. The following types of herbs may be helpful.

Emmenagogues

In this context this term denotes herbs that promote easy menstruation. If your period is often late, thick and dark, contains clots, or is sluggish, teas or tinctures of these herbs may help reduce discomfort and prevent endometriosis. Useful herbs include yarrow, feverfew, and motherwort. Many herbalists add immune-system tonics, such as ligustrum and reishi.

Yarrow is our favorite; it is easy to grow in the garden and patches grow wild all over the world. The fresh or dried flowers can be made into a tea; both the dried herb and tinctures of yarrow are widely available. If using the tincture, take 3/4 teaspoon in a little water three times daily, starting ten days before menstruation. Discontinue for the two weeks after your period ends.

Antispasmodics

For the cramps that can occur with endometriosis, herbal antispasmodics, or smooth-muscle relaxers, are helpful. Herbs in this category include cramp bark, valerian, chamomile, wild yam, false unicorn root, and California poppy.

Uterine Tonics

One of the best uterine tonics also has an effective anti-inflammatory effect: saw palmetto berry extract. The recent media attention given to saw palmetto has focused on the help it offers men with prostate difficulties, overshadowing its usefulness to women. Take two capsules in the morning, one in the evening. The herb's anti-inflammatory effects can be enhanced by using it with pumpkin seed oil or flax seed oil. To use these oils, take one teaspoon for every fifty pounds of body weight, once daily with meals.

Other effective uterine tonics include motherwort, dong quai, and red raspberry leaf. If your periods are too heavy, use red raspberry leaf.

Uterine Healers

Horsetail and plantain leaf can be especially helpful in healing endometriosis. They are thought to reduce the formation of scar tissue and keep tissues flexible. Other herbs that aid connective tissues are those containing anthocyanadins, which are also valuable antioxidants. Anthocyanadins are found in bilberries, blueberries, elderberries, green tea, hawthorn, and the seeds and skin of grapes. Gotu kola helps reduce inflammation and encourage healing. Extracts of most of these herbs are available in capsules or tablets.

Lymphatic Cleansers

One of the most important strategies for discouraging endometriosis is lymphatic cleansing. The lymphatic system, through its network of porous vessels and glands, helps the body remove toxins and infections. A massage that assists lymphatic circulation, plus herbs such as mullein, red root, and red clover that help the lymph do its job, can help prevent endometriosis from starting or progressing.

Liver Cleansers

The liver breaks down excess hormones that encourage abnormal endometrial growth. Regular liver cleansing, at least in the spring

Lymphatic System Tea

1/4 cup mullein leaves
1/4 cup red root (Ceanothus americanus)
1/4 cup red clover flowers

Blend the dried herbs together; store in an airtight container away from heat and light. Make a tea by simmering 2 teaspoons of the blend for 10 minutes in freshly boiled water. Take 1 cup of the tea daily for up to 2 weeks at a time. Take the 2-week course of this tea 3 or 4 times per year. If desired, blend equal parts of tinctures of the above herbs; take four droppersful in a little water once or twice daily for the same amount of time.

Endometriosis Tea

1 teaspoon vitex berries
1 teaspoon red clover blossoms
1 teaspoon wild yam root
1 teaspoon cramp bark
1/2 teaspoon horsetail
1/2 teaspoon red raspberry leaves
1/2 teaspoon motherwort
1 quart water

Combine herbs and water and bring to a boil. Turn down the heat and simmer gently for about 5 minutes. Remove from heat, cover, and let steep an additional 15 minutes. Strain and discard herbs; drink at least 2 cups of tea daily for 2 weeks, for a single course of treatment. This formula can also be blended from tinctures or taken in capsules.

and fall, can be effective for helping to prevent or ease symptoms of endometriosis. Good liver-cleansing herbs include the roots of dandelion, chicory, burdock, and yellow dock, and the South American herb boldo. Many commercial preparations are available.

Hormone Balancers

Vitex and black cohosh are superior herbs that help balance estrogen and progesterone. We've also found that the gamma-linolenic acid (GLA) in oils of evening primrose, currant, and borage seed may be useful for many women suffering from endometriosis. Vitex also makes a good companion herb to the emmenagogue yarrow, mentioned above.

Aromatherapy

Essential oils of some herbs may help to reduce cramping, boost the immune system, and possibly stabilize hormones; you can add these oils to massage oils and ask your massage therapist to use the mix or simply apply it yourself to moisturize the skin after bathing. Try essential oils of bergamot, sandalwood, myrrh, or helichrysum. For lymphatic massages, oils of lemon, orange, or grapefruit are helpful.

Sitz baths expose the pelvic area to alternating hot and cold water to increase blood flow. For endometriosis, we recommend sitz baths with essential oil of rosemary to increase circulation and lavender or chamomile to relax muscles and reduce inflammation.

Castor-oil packs are another time-honored remedy for relieving the pain and cramping of endometriosis. They apply moist heat and essential oils right where it hurts.

Endometriosis Massage Oil

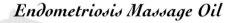

15 drops sandalwood essential oil
12 drops bergamot essential oil
8 drops lemon essential oil
8 drops myrrh essential oil
5 drops helichrysum essential oil
4 ounces vegetable oil

Combine oils. Use in abdominal massage, as a moisturizer, or add a teaspoon or two to the bath.

Endometriosis Sitz Bath

5 drops each essential oils of:
rosemary
lavender

Bring into the bathroom a tub large enough to sit in and fill it with cold water — the large plastic tubs sold at hardware and discount stores work well. Fill the bathtub with water as warm as you can stand, and add five drops each of rosemary and lavender essential oils. Sit in hot water, waist-deep or deeper, for five to ten minutes. Then switch to the cold bath for at least a minute. Repeat at least twice and up to five times, rechilling or reheating the water as necessary. For endometriosis, use the sitz bath treatment daily, if possible, for two to three weeks at a time.

Healing Castor Oil Pack

1/4 cup castor oil
8 drops lavender essential oil
small, soft cotton or flannel cloth
hot-water bottle
large towel

Preheat oven to 225 degrees. Combine lavender and castor oils, and soak the cloth in them. Fold cloth and place it in a baking dish; put in oven on center rack for about 10 minutes. Alternately, heat the prepared cloth in the microwave for about 40 seconds. Meanwhile, heat water for hot water bottle to almost boiling.

Remove the cloth from oven or microwave; it should be quite warm to the touch but not uncomfortable, so let it cool slightly if necessary. Place the folded cloth directly over the pelvic area; cover with wax paper or foil. Wrap the hot-water bottle in a large, folded towel and apply to the pack to keep in the heat. Apply the pack for a half hour to an hour daily, three to four days in a row; discontinue for the rest of the week. Resume as necessary.

CHAPTER 8

FIBROIDS AND CYSTS

*Herbalists see fibroids and cysts as places
where vital energy is stuck.*

The term "cyst" covers a multitude of conditions. For instance, if you get a splinter that resists removal, your body may form a small cyst around it, isolating it and surrounding it with fluid so that it cannot damage or infect other tissues. Simply defined, a cyst is an abnormal sac or cavity located somewhere beneath the skin and containing gas, fluid, or semisolid matter.

The vast majority of cysts cause no symptoms and are benign. But for women, two types of cysts can be troublesome: breast cysts and ovarian cysts. Uterine fibroids can cause serious problems as well.

For women, the most worrisome cysts occur in the breast, where the discovery of any lump is frightening. These cysts are almost always benign, however. The most common masses are uterine fibroids. Sometimes they are undetected; other times they lead to major surgery. Ovarian cysts can be the source of slight to debilitating pain. Understanding all three kinds of benign masses can help avoid panic or short-sighted decisions about their treatment.

NONCANCEROUS BREAST CYSTS

Breast cysts are benign sacs that are filled with fluid. Their size can vary greatly, and they may be painful. To differentiate a cyst from a solid mass which may be a tumor, a needle is inserted into the cyst and liquid removed. This causes the cyst to collapse and disappear. If this does not happen, or if there is blood in the liquid, then a mammogram and possible biopsy will be required for further diagnosis.

At least 90 percent are benign. Unlike cancerous tumors, cysts are thin and flat, usually clustered together, and often

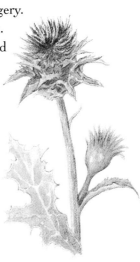

Milk Thistle

painful. Because breast cysts can obscure cancerous tumors, continue your breast self-examinations and get regular physical exams. Certainly, all breast cysts should be checked immediately.

What a Doctor Will Do

A thorough breast examination includes palpation of the entire breast and underarm areas, and sometimes the neck and abdomen. Benign cysts are typically well-defined and movable; ultrasound, a quick, harmless method, may be used to assess them. If the cysts feel suspicious to the doctor, biopsy will be recommended. A three-year European study reported in 1997 that using annual fine-needle aspiration biopsy, in which fluid is taken from the cyst with a long needle, proved nearly 100 percent accurate in detecting cancer in women with nonsuspicious cysts. Sometimes needle biopsies provide insufficient tissue for evaluation. In that case, a surgical biopsy will be performed. Breast tissue removed during biopsy will be examined for cancerous cells.

Nonsteroidal anti-inflammatory drugs (NSAIDs) such as ibuprofen or analgesics such as aspirin offer temporary relief from the pain of breast cysts but don't reduce the lumps. If pain continues, the cysts can be drained. Most doctors prefer to leave breast cysts untreated unless they become unbearable for the patient.

Another type of breast lump is fibrocystic breast disease. A number of different breast diseases are included in this category; all involve lumpy or grainy tissue in the breast. Fibrocystic breast disease can be accompanied by severe breast swelling and tenderness that varies during the menstrual cycle, decreasing after the menstrual period. These diseases are not well understood, and there are a variety of treatments that range from taking pain relievers and wearing a nighttime support bra to taking sex hormones. Persistent, painful breast cysts may be surgically removed or shrunk with hormonal drugs.

UTERINE FIBROIDS

Don't let the term "fibroid tumor" scare you. Fibroids are called tumors because they are solid masses, not because they are cancerous; almost all are benign. These slow-growing masses develop in the muscle layers of the uterine wall. Most fibroids cause no discomfort, and women are not usually aware that they are present. Others may require treatment. Fortunately, women who have fibroids may choose from several treatment options types of treatment.

Who gets fibroids? Lots of women—uterine fibroids are the most commonly found pelvic mass. The woman most likely to develop fibroids is one who has never been pregnant. Obesity, alcohol use, a high-fat diet, and a sedentary lifestyle seem to contribute to the risk of developing fibroids. Taking birth-control pills or other sources of estrogen, or a deficiency of B vitamins, may also be risk factors.

The typical woman with fibroids is between the ages of 35 and 45. Other women in her family also have them. Fibroids are rare in women under 20, but a fifth of white women and half of all African-American women over the age of 30 have them, although black women living in Africa rarely develop fibroids. Among women who have one fibroid mass, 85 percent will develop more. Some can develop 100 or more of these growths.

The Troublemakers

Not all fibroids are problem-free. For a third of women who develop them, the masses can enlarge to the size of a grapefruit. A rare fibroid can weigh up to 50 pounds, with the largest on record topping the scales at 140 pounds.

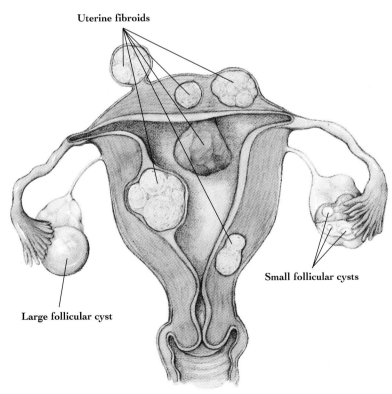

Uterine fibroids and ovarian follicular cysts

Heavy menstrual bleeding that lasts longer with each period is a warning sign of fibroids. Sometimes very severe cramps accompany fibroids, and excessive bleeding caused by them may result in extreme fatigue and even anemia.

Large fibroids may crowd surrounding organs, especially the bladder, causing pain, lots of trips to the bathroom, or retained urine. Pain in the hip or back can result from a fibroid pinching nerves in the pelvis or putting pressure on the bowel; if fibroid masses press blood vessels or kidneys, serious complications can develop. Fibroid pain typically strikes during the menstrual flow; pain at other times of the cycle probably has another source.

The Effect of Estrogen

Although the exact cause of fibroids remains unclear, they tend to form when a woman's estrogen levels are high, such as during pregnancy or while taking birth-control pills or estrogen supplements; when estrogen levels are low, as they are prior to puberty or after menopause, fibroids rarely occur. Unusually high progesterone levels may also contribute. Yet some women who have fibroids also have perfectly normal estrogen levels. Perhaps changes in the subtle balance and quality of hormones have the biggest effect, as they do in other estrogen-responsive conditions.

Fibroids may discourage fertility in several ways, such as blocking the sperm's pathway or causing the uterine lining to become so thin or undernourished that fertilized eggs cannot implant.

If pregnancy does occur, fibroids can present another set of problems. Fibroids grow more rapidly during pregnancy and may increase the chances of hemorrhage, miscarriage, or heavy postpartum bleeding. A large fibroid may obstruct delivery or interfere with uterine contractions; in such cases, the baby sometimes must be delivered by Caesarean section.

What a Doctor Will Do

A pelvic exam is usually the first step toward diagnosing fibroids. The gynecologist can easily feel a large fibroid, but small fibroid masses may require detection by other methods. Ultrasound tests can locate masses and ascertain their size, but they can't determine whether the mass is a fibroid or cancer. Occasionally magnetic resonance imaging (MRI) is used if cancer is suspected. If necessary, fibroids can also be viewed by means of a lighted scope inserted into the uterus through the cervix in a process called hysteroscopy. For direct inspection, the physician may take a small sample of uterine lining by dilation and curettage (D&C), in which the cervix is dilated and a very thin scraping of tissue removed. Most likely, the woman will be examined again in three months to determine if there is a change in the size of the fibroid, and then again every six months. Sometimes, however, surgery is the only way to distinguish a fibroid from a dangerous tumor.

For any woman diagnosed with fibroids, the most important issue is whether the mass threatens health through interference with vital organs, increased bleeding, or risk of infection. Each of these situations is potentially very serious and requires prompt action; treatment of fibroids will depend solely on the severity of symptoms.

Surgical Options

A hysterectomy—surgery to remove the uterus along with the fibroids—may be presented as your only treatment option, but this radical procedure ought to be a last resort. Among women ages 35 to 50, fibroids are the reason for 50 percent of hysterectomies. Fortunately, both women and surgeons are rethinking this once-automatic step. If no debilitating or life-threatening symptoms accompany your fibroids, your physician may be willing to take a wait-and-see approach with regular check-ups. Remember that this is your decision; the time between exams offers you a chance to try natural healing strategies.

If you choose surgery, find a surgeon who will consider alternatives to complete hysterectomy: removal of the uterus or removal of the fibroids only.

Recent European research has shown that laparoscopic surgery enables surgeons to remove fibroids while saving unaffected uterine muscle. It requires only small incisions into the abdomen. Tiny lights and surgical instruments are inserted through the incisions, and a camera provides the surgeon with the necessary interior view. Small fibroids can be removed by this method, which is far less invasive than typical abdominal surgery.

A more complicated surgery, myomectomy, removes only the fibroids while leaving the uterus intact; sometimes it can be done vaginally, without abdominal incision. More often, however, it means a major abdominal surgery, one that lasts up to several hours depending on how many fibroids the uterus holds. It may weaken the wall of the uterus, creating a risk of rupture during a later pregnancy.

Drug Treatments

An antiestrogenic drug, gonadorelin, sometimes reduces the size of fibroids by about half in three or four months, reports a 1992 British study. In a 1997 German study of 144 premenopausal women with fibroids, the drug effectively reduced the size of the masses in 90 percent of the women. Of the 43 women scheduled for hysterectomy, 29 were able to have the less serious myomectomy. Some who had planned myomectomy became eligible for the less-invasive laparoscopic surgery instead, and the fibroids of yet others became small enough to be removed vaginally. If the uterus remains after fibroid removal, the antiestrogenic drug must be continued as either injection or nasal spray. Decreased estrogen levels may result in loss of bone mass, greater susceptibility to heart disease, and other difficulties usually associated with menopause.

WHEN TO SEEK HELP FOR ABDOMINAL PAIN

Seek medical help immediately if you have the following types of lower abdominal pain:

Sudden sharp pain in lower abdomen, especially if pregnancy is a possibility

Persistent pain in the right abdomen, especially when accompanied by fever, vomiting, abdominal tenderness, and malaise

Generalized pain in the lower abdomen, especially when accompanied by fever, vaginal discharge, swelling, and abdominal tenderness

Off-and-on bursts of sharp pain in the lower abdomen, especially during intercourse, bowel movements, or other motion of the body.

OVARIAN CYSTS

Functional ovarian cysts occur as a normal part of the ovaries' job. During ovulation, an egg matures in the ovary, which protects it by forming a fluid-filled follicle sac—the cyst—around it. When the egg is mature, this sac ruptures to release it. Some women are quite aware of this process, for they experience pain, called *mittleschmerz* (German for "middle pain"), at this time. These functional cysts quickly heal.

This natural process predisposes the ovaries to produce irregular cysts as well as functional ones. Most irregular cysts resolve over time without specific intervention, but some may require surgical removal due to the potential for infection or painful pressure on adjoining areas. Ovarian cysts sometimes develop or worsen during pregnancy, due to the increased production of hormones.

Types of Ovarian Cysts

There are numerous types of abnormal ovarian cysts, but the most common occur as an outcome of incomplete ovulation or hormonal imbalance. While these cysts may cause pain and sometimes startling symptoms, they are nearly always benign and treatable.

Follicle cysts, those that are functional but do not resolve soon after the ovary releases the egg, usually get no bigger than two inches in diameter. Typically, these cysts exist quietly through a menstrual cycle or two and then rupture, causing a degree of pain. After that, they shrink.

The corpus luteum cyst, on the other hand, can grow to baseball size and cause a good deal of pain. Symptoms can also include late periods or bleeding between periods. When the cyst finally breaks, severe pain in the abdomen often radiates to the back, shoulders, and legs. This is often misdiagnosed as an ectopic, or tubal, pregnancy.

When Cysts Cause Pain

A burst cyst can cause enough pain, nausea, and weakness to warrant a trip to the emergency room. These symptoms are similar to those of even more serious emergency conditions such as an acute appendicitis, uterine or fallopian-tube infection, or ectopic pregnancy, and thus require immediate expert attention. A cyst that develops a stem and starts twisting results in intense bursts of pain; this, too, is an emergency situation. If you develop any of these symptoms, don't hesitate to seek emergency treatment.

Most frequently, however, the first sign of an ovarian cyst is mild pain or a feeling of pressure or heaviness in the lower abdomen during intercourse. Some other possible symptoms are constipation—a large cyst may press on the rectum—or frequent urges to urinate caused by pressure on the bladder.

What a Doctor Will Do

Medical treatment of ovarian cysts depends on the patient's symptoms and individual concerns. For simple cysts, draining fluid by fine-needle aspiration or other means is no more effective than leaving the cyst alone. Other cysts may require more complex treatments; laparoscopy allows the physician to assess the cyst and help you make decisions about what to do.

If symptoms indicate polycystic ovarian syndrome, a physician may suggest hormonal therapy (a combination of estrogen and progesterone), sometimes in the form of birth-control pills. Depending on the patient's individual condition, other hormone regulators may be recommended.

NATURAL HEALING

Natural medicine offers many ways of treating fibroids and cysts, most geared toward eliminating the causes as well as alleviating their symptoms. You may want to seek a health-care professional who has successfully treated the disorder in others. We've found that acupuncture is particularly effective when used with herbs and other natural healing approaches.

Women who have fibroids often see improvement with a balanced diet, loss of excess weight, and stress management. A thirty-minute walk at least three or four times a week, building up to forty-five minutes daily, increases body strength and cardiovascular health while reducing stress and helping eliminate extra pounds.

Castor-oil packs can help treat uterine fibroids and breast cysts. To prepare one, saturate a flannel cloth with castor oil and heat it in a 350-degree oven until warm. Place it over the breast or lower pelvic area and cover it with a plastic bag, a small towel, and a hot water bottle to keep it warm. The skin absorbs the castor oil's active constituents, lectins, which stimulate the local immune response to help remove cysts and tumors.

To treat breast cysts, place castor-oil packs over the breasts three or four times a week for an hour and continue for one to six months. A cabbage poultice can also be helpful. Juice one cup of raw cabbage and blend the juice with the pulp. Spread the cabbage on a small cloth or place in small muslin bag and apply over the affected area for twenty minutes at a time, several times a week, with fresh cabbage every time.

Dietary Changes

A good first line of defense against cysts is to follow a vegetarian, low-fat diet consisting of about 75 percent cooked foods, mostly grains, legumes, and vegetables; add some fish, if desired. Fruit in season and raw salads are good to eat during the warm times of the year. Use moderation with simple, refined sugar in any form, including honey and maple syrup.

Many women with breast lumps find that they can be spared biopsy and surgery if they stop drinking coffee, black or green tea, and colas, and stop eating chocolate for two or three months. Eliminating dietary caffeine helps many women; some find that their breast cysts disappear, although those 50 or older with well-established lumps may need to persist for a year or more to achieve this effect. Caffeine and related chemicals seem to stimulate overproduction of tissues that form cysts. Avoiding animal fats, hydrogenated oils, alcohol, and marijuana may also help breast lumps heal.

When treating fibroids or cysts of any kind, increase your intake of vegetables rich in carotenoids such as tomatoes, carrots, and leafy green vegetables. Eat plenty of foods rich in B vitamins, such as whole-grain products, to help keep breast cysts from swelling. Many women also benefit from increasing dietary iodine by eating more seaweed such as kelp.

Dietary Supplements

To treat fibroids, begin a daily regimen of vitamin C (1 to 2 g), beta carotene (150,000 IU), selenium (400 mcg), and zinc (30 mg). Vitamin E (400–800 IU) combined with evening primrose oil (two capsules, twice daily) seems to discourage breast cysts. We also suggest increased levels of vitamin A (up to 10,000 IU), particularly when treating breast cysts.

Herbal Healing

A useful herb for uterine fibroids is oil made from poke root. The oil may be available from an herb shop; otherwise, see your herbalist about obtaining some. Apply the oil over the tender area morning and evening. Discontinue if it causes skin irritation, and do not take the oil internally; it can cause nausea and vomiting.

When treating fibroids or cysts of any kind, we highly recommend concurrent herbal liver therapy. This organ, which cleanses toxins and excess hormones from the body, can be a powerful ally in healing. Milk thistle and burdock are the primary liver-therapy herbs.

Herbs for Breast Cysts. Breast cysts are an age-old problem, so it's not surprising that many herbs have been found to be effective against

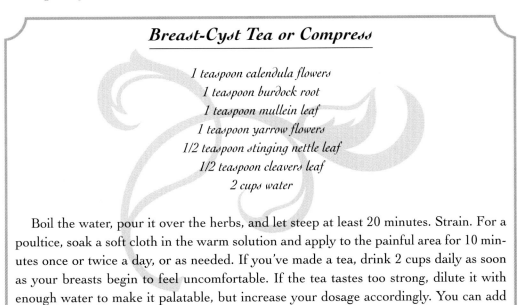

Breast-Cyst Tea or Compress

1 teaspoon calendula flowers
1 teaspoon burdock root
1 teaspoon mullein leaf
1 teaspoon yarrow flowers
1/2 teaspoon stinging nettle leaf
1/2 teaspoon cleavers leaf
2 cups water

Boil the water, pour it over the herbs, and let steep at least 20 minutes. Strain. For a poultice, soak a soft cloth in the warm solution and apply to the painful area for 10 minutes once or twice a day, or as needed. If you've made a tea, drink 2 cups daily as soon as your breasts begin to feel uncomfortable. If the tea tastes too strong, dilute it with enough water to make it palatable, but increase your dosage accordingly. You can add peppermint, wintergreen, or stevia herb to improve the taste. The herbs for breast-cyst tea can also be taken internally as tinctures or pills.

them. The nineteenth-century Swiss herbalist Father Kneipp suggested applying a poultice of calendula, horsetail, nettles, and yarrow tea to swollen breasts. To this, we add burdock, cleavers, and mullein, herbs that are traditionally used for breast swelling because they aid circulation and stimulate the lymph glands to encourage drainage. Father Kneipp also recommended drinking a tea made from the same herbs; today, they also can be taken as tinctures or pills.

Evening primrose oil may be worth a try. After starting evening primrose oil, some women notice a difference in their first menstrual cycle, but others find it takes three months or more to be effective. The oil is available only in capsules, and the effective dose varies. Most packages recommend six 500-mg capsules daily, but after results are seen, the dose can be reduced by a third or even by half. Additional herbs for breast cysts include yarrow, cleavers, and burdock to improve lymph activity.

The pain of breast cysts can be eased with warm herbal compresses placed directly where it hurts. We suggest making a strong tea of calendula, chamomile, and lavender for their anti-inflammatory and soothing properties; let the tea cool until warm. Swish a clean cotton cloth through the liquid, fold it, and apply it to the breast.

Herbs for fibroids. When herbalists get together to discuss the treatment of fibroids, they agree on one thing: These masses can be stubborn. Treatment may take several months, and sometimes the fibroids shrink,

Uterine Fibroid Tea

2 teaspoons vitex berries
1 teaspoon black cohosh
1/2 teaspoon dandelion root
1/2 teaspoon prickly ash bark
1/4 teaspoon cramp bark
1/4 teaspoon cinnamon bark
4 cups water

Combine herbs in water and bring to a boil; lower heat and simmer a few minutes. Remove from heat and steep 20 minutes. Strain and drink at least 2 cups a day. This formula or a similar one can be taken as a tincture or as pills, which many women may find practical since the formula should be continued for several months. The tincture dose is one teaspoon, three times daily, in a little water.

but do not disappear. In some difficult cases, the fibroid doesn't shrink, but does stop growing. These successes may help many women avoid surgery or hormone-altering drugs.

Vitex is an excellent herb that slows fibroid growth by normalizing hormonal balances. In some cases, it shrinks the fibroids, although this can take many months to achieve. Black cohosh also enables the body to achieve hormonal balance.

Red raspberry leaves can also reliably treat fibroids. Other traditional uterine tonics include chamomile, calendula, plantain, shepherd's purse, and St. John's wort. Herbs such as prickly ash bark, cinnamon, ginger, cleavers, and mullein improve blood and lymph circulation and support the body in its efforts to eliminate the cyst. Motherwort and dong quai can eliminate fibroids, but can also increase menstrual flow, so caution is indicated.

To treat symptoms of heavy bleeding, anemia, or severe cramps, use herbs that also treat menstrual difficulties and anemia. These include wild yam, cramp bark, and cinnamon to ease cramps, and yarrow to slow bleeding.

Fibroids, Cysts, and Traditional Chinese Medicine

According to Traditional Chinese Medicine, fibroids and cysts of any kind can be influenced by liver stagnation; bile components that are not flowing harmoniously and being eliminated from the colon collect in cysts. Bile-moving herbs for treating liver stagnation include mugwort, wormwood, artichoke leaf, and milk thistle. A highly recommended formula for treating cysts is Xiao Yao Wan, which is available in pill form in some herb stores or from practitioners of Traditional Chinese Medicine.

If a fibroid exceeds 2 centimeters in diameter, surgery is typically recommended. Traditional Chinese physicians recommend following surgery with large doses of astragalus *(huang qi)* decoction to encourage regrowth of uterine muscle.

Smaller fibroids often respond to acupuncture and herbal therapy by gradually regressing over a few months. The classic formula to accomplish this, Gui Zhi Fu Ling Tang, is a decoction of cinnamon, poria cocos, and other herbs. While a decoction is considered the best way of taking this formula, it is also available in pills, powdered concentrates, and liquid extracts.

In treating polycystic ovaries, the approach of Traditional Chinese Medicine is to increase the Yin (female hormones) and bring the Yang (male hormones) into balance. Because practitioners of this type of medicine interpret and treat the condition in several ways, the patient is usually asked to record her temperature upon awakening each morning for a month. This information enables the practitioner to determine if the condition is one of "high temperature" or "low temperature". Upon diagnosis, the practitioner will design a specific therapy that is likely to include acupuncture.

Herbal therapy often accompanies acupuncture treatment and may include rehmannia root, scrophularia root, dendrobium stem, and asparagus root. To break down the cysts, herbs that eliminate stagnation and masses are used; these include roots of red peony, tree peony, and red Chinese sage root.

Aromatherapy

A quick compress made by adding the following essential oils and tinctures of herbs to warm water promotes circulation and healing for breast cysts.

For uterine fibroids, add five drops of essential oil of lavender to a castor-oil pack. Place the pack over the uterine area two to four times weekly, keeping it warm. Also use sitz baths containing several drops of rosemary, lavender, or juniper essential oils to encourage circulation in the lower abdomen. Acupuncture and lymph massage can accelerate the effects of these treatments.

Breast Compress with Essential Oils

1/2 teaspoon calendula flower tincture
10 drops lavender essential oil
3 drops chamomile essential oil
1 cup warm water

Combine ingredients in a shallow bowl. Swish a small, soft cloth in the solution. Wring cloth out over the bowl and fold into several layers. Immediately place over swollen breast for 5 to 10 minutes. Run another cloth under cold water and wring out. Exchange the warm compress for the cold one and leave on about 2 minutes. Alternate the cloths back and forth a few times. This compress can also be made with 1/2 cup each of lavender and chamomile tea instead of the essential oils.

CHAPTER 9

VAGINAL INFECTIONS

Yeast and other bacterial infections can be a signal that the body is out of balance. Relieving symptoms is important — but so is correcting the imbalance.

Most women have experienced at least one vaginal infection, and many have had several. Typical symptoms include irritation, redness, and swelling of the vulvar area, along with an unusual discharge. The color, odor, and type of discharge give clues about the troublesome organism; treatment follows identification of the culprit. Yeast infections associated with *Candida albicans* occur frequently, but organisms such as the protozoan *Trichomonas vaginalis* and unfriendly bacteria, among them *Gardnerella vaginalis*, cause similar symptoms.

If you notice a slight, painless, but increased vaginal discharge, you can probably restore balance and reduce symptoms using the natural methods described in this chapter. If the discharge persists or becomes painful or heavy, or occurs with pelvic pain or fever, seek the help of a qualified health-care practitioner or physician.

HOW INFECTIONS HAPPEN

The internal walls of the healthy vagina continuously produce cleansing secretions that maintain a mildly acidic environment and inhibit infections. Normal vaginal discharge varies in color and consistency because it responds to changing hormonal levels during the menstrual cycle.

Many observant women are familiar with their changes in vaginal discharge. As menses ends, hormone levels drop and vaginal discharge often becomes minimal. During the next ten days to two weeks, the discharge likely becomes increasingly white or yellow and creamy as hormone

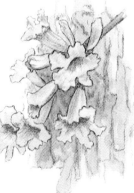

Pau d'arco

levels increase; at ovulation, the discharge becomes transparent and stringy, forming a "bridge" from the vaginal floor to the cervix that helps sperm cells enter the cervical canal to reach and fertilize egg cells. After ovulation the mucus is again white or yellow and scanty.

Any other changes in discharge should be promptly investigated, for the vagina can provide a perfect environment for unwanted organisms. Warm, moist, and dark, it contains a range of nutrients in the form of mucus, sugars, and shed epithelial cells. The vaginal environment can be disrupted by tampons, vaginal creams, sprays, birth-control gels, IUDs, douches, and traces of fecal matter.

Sexual intercourse can introduce infections and disrupt the vagina's protective acidity. Many pathogens and toxins can ride in the seminal fluid of an unhealthy partner. In addition, seminal fluid is alkaline. Frequent exposure to it disrupts vaginal pH and increases chances of infection. Condoms offer a measure of protection.

Normal vaginal acidity may also be disrupted by heavy intake of sugar and refined carbohydrates. Diabetic women are also at risk, as are pregnant women or those undergoing hormone-replacement therapy or taking birth-control pills. Post-menopausal levels of estrogen and progesterone encourage some vaginal infections.

> *If your symptoms are accompanied by fever, pain, or an altered menstrual cycle, promptly seek professional help.*

Antibiotics are the nemesis of the vagina's natural protective flora. These drugs indiscriminately destroy infectious and friendly bacteria alike, creating imbalances such as the overgrowth of *Candida albicans,* or yeast infection. Even if antibiotics stop infection, they do nothing for the overall health of the reproductive organs. For infections we feel that antibiotics should be used only for severe cases such as pelvic inflammatory disease (PID). When it is necessary to use them, we urge that you do so with the support of a healthy diet, herbs that help the body restore immune balance, and probiotics such as live-culture yogurt to help restore the normal flora. Your doctor may prescribe an antiyeast vaginal cream along with the antibiotics, especially if you mention that you are prone to yeast infections.

The three most common vaginal infections include trichomoniasis (overgrowth of the protozoan *Trichomonas vaginalis*), yeast infections (overgrowth of *Candida albicans*), and bacterial vaginosis (associated primarily with *Gardnerella vaginalis*). Together, these organisms are responsible for about 90 percent of all vaginal infections.

Yeast Infections

Yeast infection is associated with the common organism *Candida albicans* and a few of its relatives; all normally reside in the intestines and vagina. These bacteria cause trouble only when their populations get out of hand, producing an irritating discharge accompanied by swelling, itching, and redness.

Several factors promote yeast infections. Antibiotics are especially notorious and probably a major reason that the frequency of yeast infections has more than doubled since the late 1960s. Women who have allergies also seem more likely to develop yeast infections.

Anything that increases blood-sugar levels can promote yeast overgrowth; examples include uncontrolled diabetes, pregnancy, or eating sugary foods regularly. The use of vaginal sponges and IUDs raises blood sugar. High estrogen levels increase sugar levels and can also help candida cells attach to the vaginal wall to form colonies. Women are more susceptible to candida overgrowth the week before menstruation. Wearing tight-fitting and/or synthetic undergarments, bathing in chlorinated pools or hot tubs, using harsh soap, and douching frequently also contribute to infection. Candida find it easier to proliferate if you are under stress or physically weakened.

Candida cells take two forms—the normal round cell and a long, thin, rapidly growing and budding form. The thin cells aggressively pry apart the cells of the vaginal walls and invade deeper tissues, creating more severe symptoms of thick vaginal discharge, yeast odor, and itching of the vulva.

A SYMPTOM, NOT A CAUSE

The organism candida, or yeast, is usually present in the healthy vagina, where it co-exists harmoniously with other organisms. When the vaginal environment is disrupted, however, candida grows rapidly and can become a problem. Consequently, the organism is not the cause of infection so much as an opportunist willing to participate in the entire process of disease.

Look at it this way: The infection is simply a signal that the body is out of balance. Killing the offending organisms relieves symptoms and resolves the infection, but the imbalances that allowed the infectious organism to build its numbers remain.

While a natural approach to healing aims to ease the same symptoms, it focuses on identifying and correcting this fundamental imbalance. It requires greater self-awareness and trust in the body's intrinsic power to heal itself.

Can yeast infections be transmitted sexually? Professional opinions vary, and these infections are not classified as a sexually transmitted disease. To be safe, however, your male partner can seek treatment — particularly if your infections recur without explanation. Some clinical studies show that candida can be cultured from the genitals of 5 to 25 percent of male partners of infected women.

When Yeast Infections Become Chronic

Some women have recurring, stubborn bouts of yeast infection that may be related to a genetically determined weak immune response or to a hypersensitive or allergic reaction to the organism. Candida can invade other parts of the body; recently, many special diets, herbal cures, and nutritional supplements have been promoted to treat this condition.

Many women who receive a diagnosis of systemic candida infection may instead suffer from adrenal fatigue, chronic fatigue syndrome, food allergies, environmental sensitivities, fibromyalgia, or other conditions arising from overwork, stress, and poor diet. True chronic candida infection usually indicates a weakened immune system, a diagnosis that calls for further testing.

Candida cells

Those who have chronic vaginal yeast infections can be prone to systemic yeast infections and should carefully follow a balanced, low-sugar, whole-foods diet. A powerful herbal and nutritional supplement program can also help.

Bacterial Vaginosis

The second most common vaginal infection, bacterial vaginosis, is usually associated with the bacteria *Gardnerella vaginalis*. The bacteria is present in the vaginas of 50 to 60 percent of healthy women; bacterial vaginosis is diagnosed when *Gardnerella* increases in tandem with:

- increased numbers of anaerobic organisms such as *Peptostreptococcus* and *Bacteroides*
- pH higher than 4.5
- decreased numbers of *Lactobacillus*.

Bacterial vaginosis is particularly worrisome because the bacteria can easily infect the uterus and fallopian tubes, leading to pelvic inflammatory disease (PID). This painful condition can damage fertility and reproductive organs. Infected pregnant women are more likely to face preterm delivery than healthy women and more likely to contract endometrial infection after giving birth.

Gardnerella is believed to be sexually transmitted, but its exact causes are unknown. Certainly an infected woman's sexual partner should be treated.

Trichomoniasis

Caused by one-celled protozoans called *trichomonas*, trichomoniasis is common and rarely serious. Yet it's far more unpleasant than a yeast infection and more difficult to cure. It produces a thick, yellowish, frothy discharge (sometimes with blood), and swollen, inflamed genitals that burn and itch. By inflaming the urethra and bladder, trichomoniasis causes frequent, burning urination. The organism prefers an alkaline environment, a natural vaginal condition that becomes more pronounced around menstruation. Up to 20 percent of women in their reproductive years will suffer through this infection at least once.

This microorganism is transmitted both sexually and nonsexually; 2.5 to 3 million cases occur annually in the United States. Infected men rarely show symptoms, although they can transmit trichomoniasis; 60 percent of infected women can also be symptom-free. Non-sexual transfer sometimes occurs because the organism can survive on moist surfaces like damp towels or bathing suits and in swimming pools and hot tubs. Trichomonas dies quickly when dried out, so dry toilet seats or towels present no danger.

COMMON VAGINAL INFECTIONS

Organism(s)	Appearance	Odor	Notes
Candida	Curdy, white, cottage cheese-like	No smell or a "yeasty" one	Most common; often occurs during pregnancy or after taking antibiotics or high-estrogen birth-control pills
Gardnerella	Thin, gray or greenish; pH is 4.5 or higher	Foul or fishy	Second most common infection
Trichomonas	Copious, yellow or greenish, frothy, pH of 6 to 7	Foul or fishy	Can occur with bacterial vaginosis; is usually sexually transmitted; can be symptomless

What a Doctor Will Do

A gynecologist will first take your health history to determine risk for vaginal infections; answers to all questions, even those about sexual partners, are confidential. The pelvic examination will include the vulva, vagina, and cervix; with probing pressure, the physician will evaluate the uterus and ovaries for tenderness and inflammation. After examining a sample of vaginal discharge with a microscope, the doctor may send it to a lab for culture; additional tests may be done to determine the organism responsible for the infection. A urine sample may also be taken to determine whether the infection has moved up the urinary tract.

Doctors initially treat uncomplicated yeast infections with an antifungal: nystatin (Mycostatin or Nilstat), miconazole (Monistat), clotrimazole (Gyne-Lotrimin), butaconazole 2-percent cream, or terconazole suppositories. Prescription-strength or over-the-counter forms may be recommended. Some doctors suggest boric acid powder in a 00-size capsule as a vaginal suppository.

For trichomoniasis, doctors typically prescribe Flagyl. Creams or suppositories of Betadine or Trichotine may also be prescribed. Your sexual partner should be treated simultaneously. Flagyl is associated with cancer and birth defects in animals; it upsets digestion, reduces white blood-cell production, and should not be used during pregnancy

ANTIBIOTICS FOR VAGINAL INFECTIONS: THE RISKS, THE BENEFITS

Many drugs prescribed for vaginal infections can cause increased vulvar and vaginal irritation, redness, itching, and even discharge, especially if you are sensitive to them. Headaches, body aches, and abdominal symptoms sometimes occur. Many of these drugs have not been proven safe for use during pregnancy and should not be taken during the first trimester. Many should not be used concurrently with alcoholic beverages. Caution is always advised when you have a pre-existing liver condition.

Read the instructions carefully, including all the contraindications and side effects, and get information from your doctor. If in doubt, consult your pharmacist and/or review the drug in the current *Physicians Desk Reference* (PDR), available at most libraries and many bookstores. In most cases, especially mild or chronic ones, natural remedies offer additional health benefits and fewer side effects.

or breast feeding. Side effects include nausea, diarrhea, headaches and a metallic taste in the mouth. Avoid alcohol if taking Flagyl.

Bacterial vaginosis treatments may include Flagyl, Cleocin, or Metrogel. The latter two are typically prepared as vaginal creams.

NATURAL HEALING

Healthy Habits

Many natural strategies can assist the prevention and healing of vaginal infections—from those that are common and annoying to those that are rare.

First, keep your immune system active and strong with healthy diet, daily exercise, regular stretching, and sound sleep. Because stress and overwork weaken the immune system, try to reduce them by adjusting your work schedule or making time for activities that reduce stress. Positive, supportive relationships help, too.

Be sure to get plenty of exercise and fresh air. Because the perception of stressful events and relationships influences immune response, you may want to improve your ways of coping with stress, perhaps by seeking counseling, participating in a spiritually oriented group, or reading inspirational books.

If you now wear tight or synthetic underwear, switch to cotton with a gentle fit. Synthetic fabrics retain moisture and heat while reducing air circulation in the vaginal area; unfriendly organisms thrive in these conditions, while beneficial bacteria decline.

> ## IF YOU'RE TAKING ANTIBIOTICS...
>
> Here are three easy-to-find, natural remedies that can help these pharmaceutical drugs accomplish their task and minimize their side effects.
>
> **A probiotic supplement** such as *Lactobacillus acidophilus* restores beneficial microorganisms to the digestive tract.
>
> **Echinacea** stimulates the immune system. Take four droppersful of a tincture two or three times daily.
>
> **Milk-thistle extract** helps your liver. Take 300 to 400 milligrams in tablets or capsules daily.

Keep the vulva free of odor-causing bacteria. Daily washing eliminates fecal matter that can contaminate the area. Using clean water during a shower is often sufficient, but a solution of apple cider vinegar or a light soap is also effective. Urine residue may actually help prevent infections; it contains urea, allantoin (an active compound in plantain and comfrey), and other natural antibiotics.

Too-frequent douching upsets the balance of the vagina's microflora. Some gynecologists believe that any douching can upset the vaginal balance or spread infection into the uterus, but we have never known this to be a problem. If you douche, do it right: Make sure that the water flow is not too forceful by suspending the bag no higher than shoulder level. Use a douche to treat an occasional infection, but not as a daily or even weekly freshener. If you use a commercial preparation, try substituting this gentle recipe:

The Apple Cider Vinegar Douche

To treat minor vaginal infections, use this natural douche of unpasteurized, diluted apple cider vinegar to normalize the vagina's acidity and thus prevent proliferation of destructive microorganisms.

2 tablespoons unpasteurized apple cider vinegar
2 cups of warm water

Pour solution into douche bag or bulb. Allow the flow from the nozzle to gently rinse the vagina. During an infection, douche once a day, but to maintain health, douche only once or twice a month.

Dietary Changes

Women with stubborn, recurring infections or overgrowth of candida should try a whole-foods diet that excludes all sugar, even fruits. For acute, feverish infection, perhaps with rash, emphasize cooling foods such as fresh vegetables and vegetable juices. For chronic infection, a diet strong in legumes, whole grains, fish, poultry, and lightly cooked vegetables is best.

Probiotics: The Friendly Bacteria

When taking antibiotics for an infection, it is important to reduce their impact on your digestive tract, liver, and immune system. To replenish the friendly bacteria in the colon after antibiotic use, we recommend probiotic supplements such as acidophilus, usually found in the refrigerator section of natural products stores. Select capsules that contain about one billion viable organisms each; take two capsules with breakfast and one with dinner for a month or two. For chronic vaginal infections, take the supplements continuously.

Eating yogurt helps; we recommend eight ounces daily. Look for "live cultures" on the label; some manufacturers heat yogurt during processing, killing the friendly microorganisms. We've also found that live-culture, plain yogurt added to a douche reduces unwanted pathogens, especially yeast, and soothes irritated areas. Studies have found that a live strain of *Lactobacillus acidophilus* works well, but avoid the strains *L. bulgaris* and *L. thermophilus;* they're not effective for vaginal infection.

Other Foods to Add

Garlic is a potent antibacterial, antifungal, and antiviral herb, so if you love it—and those who kiss you don't mind—here's your excuse to indulge. Eat two or three cloves per day, or take a powdered supplement.

Two other common spices—turmeric and ginger—can be added to foods to help support the liver. If you suspect that an overabundance of estrogen may be a culprit in your infection, see the Dietary Strategies section in the PMS chapter for foods that help regulate estrogen production.

Herbal Healing

Fortunately for infection sufferers, many herbal remedies can help. Herbal compounds can ease the pain and itch of inflammation, fight infectious organisms, and assist the body's natural defenses.

Immune Boosters

Many infections respond to a one-two punch: internal formulas that contain immune-stimulating herbs, and herbal preparations that kill or inhibit the pathogens. Below are some potent immune-boosting herbs.

Echinacea. You've probably heard of this herb as one of the first-line defenses against cold and flu symptoms. Its immune-stimulating properties are also helpful against many vaginal infections and sexually transmitted diseases. It can be taken internally as a tea, tincture, or pill. You also can apply a weak tea of the herb directly to the infected vagina.

In a study of a commercial echinacea product, Echinacin, recurring yeast infections fell from 60 percent to 16 percent when echinacea was taken orally along with econazol nitrate, an antifungal drug. Echinacea can be used along with berberine-containing herbs to stimulate immune activity for clearing an infection.

DIETARY SUPPLEMENTS FOR INFECTIONS
During an infection, whether it is sexually transmitted or not, it can be beneficial to increase the daily dose of certain vitamins.
Vitamin A: 25,000 units at first, then 5,000 to 10,000 IU
Beta carotene: 100,000 to 200,000 IU
Vitamin C: 2 grams twice daily
Vitamin B complex: as directed on the product label
Zinc: 15 mg daily
Vitamin E: 400 IU daily
Folic acid: 10 mg daily for three months, then 2.5 mg daily for one year

Other immune stimulants that may be helpful include wild indigo root *(Baptisia tinctoria)*, the Chinese herb isatis, poke root, osha, and yerba mansa.

Women's Anti-Infection Tea

2 teaspoons echinacea root
1 teaspoon Oregon grape root
1 teaspoon vitex seeds
3 cups water

Combine herbs and water in a pan and bring to a boil for a few minutes, turn down the heat, and simmer gently 15 minutes. Remove from heat and steep 20 minutes. Strain out herbs. Drink 3 to 4 cups daily.

Immune Support for Stubborn Infections

If an infection lasts for more than a month or recurs often, avoid echinacea. An overworked immune system needs support, not more stimulation. Instead, for recurring or stubborn vaginal infections, use a deep-acting herbal program that supports and strengthens immune function.

Try astragalus, ligustrum, shiitake, reishi, nettles, and burdock root in tea, capsules, or tablets for about three months; it takes time to rebuild and restore immune strength. Nine months of consistent treatment nearly always result in benefits.

These immune-strengthening herbs also can be simmered for forty-five minutes, cooled, and strained. You can use the broth in soups or stews. Add nourishing green vegetables, a little fish or chicken if desired, and adzuki or mung beans for added protein.

Liver Support Herbs

To support the liver in cleansing the body of wastes from infections or viruses, or to strengthen it during and after antibiotic use, milk thistle is nearly always recommended, in doses of 200 to 400 milligrams per day. Here are other liver-boosting herbs you may wish to try.

- Schisandra berry: two cups daily of tea or four capsules of the powder twice daily.
- Dandelion root and burdock root tea; take two cups daily. Alternately, take four capsules of this combination twice daily.

Antibacterial Preparations

Correctly used, certain herbs can eliminate vaginal infection while improving your overall health. These herbs, prepared in douches or suppositories, attack pathogens directly. They're the second "punch" in an effective herbal program to fight infection. They are usually effective within a week or so. Some persistent infections may take two weeks to resolve. If you see no improvement after that time, consult a qualified health practitioner.

Herbs containing the alkaloid berberine. Goldenseal, barberry, Oregon grape root, and the Chinese herbs coptis and phellodendron help eliminate most vaginal pathogens.

A douche of phellodendron bark, also known as *huang bai,* treats trichomoniasis effectively. Tablets of berberine sulfate *(huang lian su),* can also be found in Chinese pharmacies or natural products stores. Under the advice of your herbalist or health-care practitioner, take one or two

---

Berberine Douche for Trichomoniasis

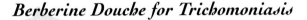

An effective douche can be made using coptis, phellodendron, Oregon grape root, barberry, or goldenseal.

1 to 1½ tablespoons of coarsely ground or chopped herb
1 cup of water

Simmer the herb and water for 15 minutes, remove from heat, and steep for 20 minutes. Let cool. If desired, make enough of the preparation to last for 4 days and store in the refrigerator.

Caution: Do not use during pregnancy.

Agrimony Douche for Trichomoniasis

1 tablespoon agrimony
1 cup water

Simmer the herb for 15 minutes, then let cool. Strain; use the tea twice daily as a douche.

tablets orally morning and evening, or insert one tablet in the vagina, morning and evening. The preparation is generally safe, but excessive amounts or use for more than ten days can produce side effects such as digestive upset.

Caution: Under no conditions use berberine or berberine-containing herbs during pregnancy.

Garlic. An effective antibacterial and antifungal, garlic destroys candida and improves most vaginal infections. Eating two or three cloves of garlic daily works wonders.

Rosemary, thyme, and lavender. Any of these aromatic herbs, made into a weak tea and used as a douche, acts powerfully against bacteria; thyme and rosemary are the strongest.

Agrimony. This herb can be purchased in natural food stores or herb shops. In Chinese medicine, the herb is known as *xian he cao*. A strong douche is effective against trichomonas.

Quick Yogurt Douche

This preparation helps restore beneficial microorganisms.

3 drops lavender essential oil
3 drops tea tree essential oil
3 cups warm water
2 heaping tablespoons plain yogurt with live Lactobacillus acidophilus *cultures*

Combine ingredients in a douche bag. Mix well. Use the douche once daily for up to seven days. For vaginitis or cervical ulceration, add wild indigo root to the

Gentle Herbal Douche

This preparation is for mild or moderate infections.

1 tablespoon rosemary, thyme, or lavender
1 cup water

Heat water just to boiling. Pour over the herbs; steep covered for 10 minutes. Strain and let cool; use as a daily douche for a week or so.

Herbal douches can also help ease the symptoms of candida or other infections. Teas of slippery elm or marshmallow root can be used as main ingredients in a douche to soothe irritated tissues. Mildly astringent herbs can help dry discharge caused by an infection. These include red raspberry leaf, strawberry leaf, and willow leaves; make a weak tea, then use as you would other douches.

External Applications

For irritation, redness, and itching of the vulva, apply a cream or light salve containing soothing herbs such as aloe vera gel, calendula, chamomile, or plantain leaf. You can add one part aloe vera gel to one part calendula or chamomile cream your-self. Apply to irritated membranes as needed. Avoid creams that contain perfumes or essential oils.

Aloe Vera

Specific Remedies: Yeast Infections

For candida or yeast infections, turn to black walnut, pau d'arco, tea tree, rosemary, thyme, and garlic. The inner bark of pau d'arco, a South American tree, contains compounds that inhibit candida. Pau d'arco can be brewed into tea by simmering one teaspoon of the herb in a cup of water for fifteen minutes; drink two or three cups daily. Pau d'arco combines well with other herbs.

The Yeast-Fighter

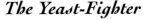

1/4 cup pau d'arco inner bark
1/4 cup black walnut hulls
1/4 cup rosemary herb
1/4 cup nettle herb
1 tablespoon licorice root, coarsely ground
Water to cover

Simmer the herbs for 5 minutes in a covered pot; steep for 15 minutes. Drink 1 cup morning, afternoon, and evening. Use 1 cup as a douche at room temperature, morning and evening, for the first few days, then once a day for another 5 days or so. Continue for one or two days after symptoms disappear.

Aromatherapy

A helpful essential oil for vaginal infection is derived from *Eucalyptus polybractea*, or blue malle. If this particular eucalyptus is not available, do not replace it with another eucalyptus. Instead, use lavender or tea tree essential oil.

Diluted essential oils are good preventives for women who get frequent infections, especially after intercourse. Lavender essential oil is particularly effective in destroying candida, and it smells good, too. Tea tree oil suppositories are available in some natural products stores.

Lavender Vaginal Oil

¼ cup vegetable oil
¼ teaspoon lavender essential oil

Combine ingredients well. Apply daily to vagina with fingers, or apply ½ teaspoon to the end of a tampon end and insert. If desired, use as a vaginal lubricant. (If you are using condoms, substitute glycerin-based extracts for the essential oil.)

CHAPTER 10

URINARY TRACT INFECTIONS

Some women react to these infections much more severely than others. Some never get them at all. Herbs and healing foods can be just as effective as medical solutions for healing and protecting the urinary tract.

After flu and vaginal infections, infections of the bladder and urinary tract are the most common infections among women. Up to 5 percent of women's doctor visits are motivated by symptoms of urinary tract infection. These problems occur more frequently among older women.

The symptoms include painful and frequent urination, the urge to urinate although the bladder is nearly empty, and pressure and pain in the lower pelvis. They can be unpleasant and persist for days or longer. Fever may accompany the infection, and blood or pus may be found in the urine. Urinary tract infections often recur, sometimes several times a year; researchers studying a group of 60 women experiencing their first urinary tract infections found that nearly 30 percent had a recurrence over the next 18 months. The same researchers studied a group of 106 women with a history of urinary tract infections and found that nearly 83 percent had a recurrence.

Most urinary tract infections are associated with the ubiquitous *E. coli,* a bacteria normally found in the bowel. Typically, these bacteria also live on the perineum, the area between the anus and the vagina. Recurring urinary tract infections are always associated with the increased presence of bacteria around the vaginal opening. From the vagina, it is a short distance to the opening of the urethra.

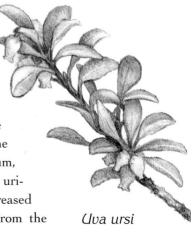

Uva ursi

Women experience urinary tract infections more frequently than men due to a simple structural difference: The urethra, which conducts urine from the bladder to the outside of the body, is three times longer in men than women. Thus, bacteria can easily travel the short distance to the female bladder to establish infection; then bacterial by-products stimulate the body's immune responses, producing inflammation and swelling.

Some women react to these infections much more strongly than others. Some women never get them in the first place. Why? Scientists don't know yet, but we believe diet, immune status, and hygiene are factors. Repeated bladder infections can endanger health. Chronic bacterial overgrowth and infection of the bladder can occur without symptoms in 5 to 7 percent of women of childbearing age, and up to 15 percent of women over 65. These bacteria can also travel from the bladder up the ureters to infect the kidneys and cause inflammation. Kidney infection (pyelonephritis) can occur without signs or symptoms and remain undetected until it causes major damage and even kidney failure.

If you have fever, chills, nausea, and vomiting, with pain under the lower ribs, you may have a kidney infection. This calls for a trip to the doctor for a diagnosis, because kidney damage can occur if left untreated.

WHAT A DOCTOR WILL DO

A doctor will likely evaluate your symptoms and palpate the area over your bladder (right above the pubic bone) for sensitivity or pain. A urine sample will be taken; diagnosis is based on the presence of white blood cells and bacteria in the urine. Sometimes a quick screening is done using a dipstick in a urine sample, which gives a rapid measurement of the presence of white blood cells.

Antibiotics will be prescribed immediately—most likely sulfonamides (Sulfisoxazole), ampicillin, nitrofurantoin, tetracycline, cephalexin, cephradine, or quinolones—for three days to two weeks. These drugs often successfully eliminate bacteria from the bladder, urethra, and kidney, but infections can recur. If you do not take the drugs for the full time prescribed, the bacteria are more likely to recur, and by then they may have become drug-resistant.

RISK FACTORS FOR URINARY TRACT INFECTIONS

Increased sexual activity

Weakened immune function

Poor hygiene

Other vaginal illnesses

Vaginal bacterial imbalance

Exposure to allergenic foods such as wheat, eggs, dairy products

Condom use

Spermicide use

Anatomical abnormalities

Antibiotics destroy beneficial bacteria in the colon, vagina, and mouth, making other infections, especially yeast infections, more likely to occur. They can also lead to digestive disturbances such as decreased assimilation of nutrients, nausea, gas, and intestinal discomfort. Many antibiotics stress the liver and kidneys.

Three-day antibiotic treatments are becoming more common. This strategy may reduce the drugs' impact on overall health but is less effective at eliminating infection. A follow-up urine test to make sure the infection is gone may be a wise choice.

Natural Healing

Healthy Habits

Vigorous, sweaty exercise helps your body eliminate toxic wastes without burdening the kidneys. If you don't perspire, these toxins must be eliminated by the bowels, kidneys, and bladder. Saunas and vigorous skin brushing with a dry brush or loofa can also enhance elimination.

Careful attention to hygiene around the anus and sex organs is essential. Using a tea tree soap in daily showers to cleanse the perineum and afterward splashing fresh water over the vulva and vaginal opening can help disrupt bacterial colonies. Avoid scented toilet tissues, vaginal sprays or perfumes, and bubble baths; these can cause allergic reactions.

Dietary Changes

Diet and stress factors can have a powerful effect on whether an individual will get urinary tract infections. To avoid them, we recommend a whole-foods diet low in processed sugars, coffee and other caffeine-containing drinks, and alcohol.

Base the diet on rice and beans, with fish, chicken, and turkey if desired. Include soothing foods such as barley soup, okra, and flax seed, as well as kidney-strengthening foods like adzuki beans, yams, burdock root, winter squash, and fish. Eat most foods at room temperature or warmer, and avoid cold foods.

Dietary Supplements

We recommend adding the following vitamins and nutrients to your diet, especially if they are in short supply in your regular foods.

• Vitamin C, 1 to 4 grams daily, spread over the course of the day

- Flavonoid-rich herbs such as orange peel, hawthorn, and rose hips; take up to 500 mg daily to reduce inflammation

- Antioxidants such as grape-seed extract, 200 to 400 mg daily, to reduce inflammation and tissue damage

- Vitamin E, 400 to 800 IU a day

- Flax seed oil, one tablespoon for every fifty pounds of body weight. You can also sprinkle the oil on food or take it in capsules

- Acidophilus supplements.

Herbal Remedies

Herbs are the ideal remedy for preventing and healing urinary tract infections. They do not have the side effects of antibiotics, yet are often just as effective, especially when coupled with dietary changes such as reducing sugar intake. An effective herbal program for urinary tract

THE CRANBERRY SOLUTION

Cranberry juice or a powder made from the juice is certainly the most widely recommended natural remedy for urinary tract infections. Cranberry has gained wide acceptance in natural medicine and modern medicine alike, partly because definitive scientific studies say it works, but also because it really does.

Researchers have concluded that when the juice's organic acids pass through the urinary tract, they increase acidity and discourage bacterial growth. The acids also interfere with the bacteria's ability to attach to the bladder wall and cause infection. Another phenolic compound, hippuric acid, is formed from benjoic acid when the juice passes through the digestive tract. This acid can inhibit pathogenic *E. coli.*

Cranberry can be used simply as a juice taken between meals; drink a glassful several times a day, up to a quart. We prefer the straight juice, lightly sweetened. Supplements in capsules are also available.

In one study, half of a group of 153 women each consumed 300 milliliters of cranberry beverage for 6 months. In the juice drinkers, pathogenic bacteria counts were about half as high as they were in women who drank a placebo.

Cranberry may not be the best remedy for healing an acute infection, but it can be begun as soon as the first symptoms are felt and continued for two months to prevent a recurrence. If you are prone to recurring infections, try using the supplement and the other herbs and vitamins described in this chapter continuously for up to three months. Then take a break for several months.

infections should include representatives of several groups of herbs. Select two to five herbs from each group, depending on what is available to you and what you know works well with your body.

Soothing, Demulcent Herbs

This group of herbs includes those whose water-soluble mucilage reduces inflammation.

Marshmallow root can be used as the basis of many soothing teas and tinctures.

Corn silk is the long thready strands of the corn ear's female pistils. A traditional remedy for soothing and cooling the urinary tract, it is included in many urinary formulas that can be purchased at herb or natural products stores. Follow the manufacturer's directions.

Plantain leaf contains a high percentage of mucilage and the compound allantoin, which helps speed the healing process and prevent scarring. Plantain is a common weed worldwide; when fresh, it also contains a strong antibiotic compound, aucubin. Fresh plantain leaves can be harvested and put through a juicer or blended with barley water to make a soothing and healing drink for the urinary tract.

Flax seed contains abundant mucilage. You can brew a tea using one teaspoon of flax seeds for each cup of water. Simmer for five minutes and let the mixture steep for fifteen or twenty minutes. Drink up to three or four cups daily.

Antibacterial Herbs

Pipsissewa, abundant in the Pacific Northwest mountains, is a Native American remedy for urinary infections and irritation. Highly effective for soothing and mildly disinfecting the urinary tract, it can be used as a light decoction or as a liquid tincture.

Usnea contains several antibiotic compounds that kill bacteria. In our experience, it is one of the most effective herbs for preventing or curing urinary tract infections. Use it in tincture form because the antibacterial compounds are poorly soluble in water. One teaspoon of the liquid tincture in a little water several times a day for ten days constitutes one course; up to three courses can be taken with three days off between courses.

Uva ursi means "bear-grapes." Bears are believed to enjoy the plant's red berries. The young tender tips of

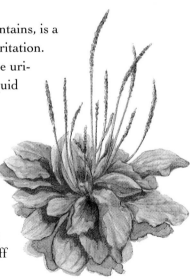

Plaintain

branches are harvested for liquid tinctures and teas. The plant has demulcent, astringent, and antibacterial properties and is renowned for healing chronic urinary tract infections. Decoctions or tinctures can be taken for seven to ten days.

Goldenseal, barberry, coptis, and **Oregon grape root** contain berberine, an antibacterial alkaloid. Teas or tinctures of these herbs, or pills of refined berberine extracted from the Chinese herb coptis, are available from natural products stores or herb shops. Take two tablets morning and evening for up to a week, preferably on the advice of your acupuncturist or herbalist.

Myrrh, in tincture form, can be added to formulas for its antibiotic and astringent properties. Follow the manufacturer's instructions on dosage.

Propolis is a bee product made from the resins of cottonwood trees. The tincture is highly antibacterial. Take two to three droppersful with other herbs in a little water, several times daily.

Juniper berry liquid extract or tea is a traditional remedy for preventing and healing urinary tract infections. Juniper berry tea is a good preventative when used for a week or two as a light decoction. Two or three cups can be taken daily. Do not, however, take the essential oil internally.

Immune-boosting Herbs

Immune stimulants include echinacea, osha, and wild indigo root.

Immune tonics such as astragalus, ligustrum, shiitake, and reishi can be used for several months up to a year to help support the immune system.

Bladder tonics include saw palmetto, nettle leaves and root, goldenrod, kava kava, horsetail, and the Chinese herb cornus fruit. These herbs stimulate the flow of blood and nutrients to the urinary tract.

All of the above herbs can be found in tincture form; many can be found in capsules or tablets. You may find that the easiest way to take them in combination is to purchase a commercial formula that combines several. Be sure to continue taking the tonic herbs for three to five weeks after the acute phase of an infection is over.

Additional Helpful Herbs

Aquaretics include herbs such as dandelion leaf and parsley root that increase the output of urine to help flush out bacteria and toxic waste products. Both herbs can be eaten fresh or brewed for tea.

Flavonoid-rich herbs can help reduce the heat of infection and calm inflammation. Teas of hawthorn fruit, rose hips, and orange peel are excellent sources. Commercial products in capsule or tablet form containing these herbs are also widely available, sometimes blended with vitamin C.

Antioxidants help prevent tissue damage by mopping up dangerous free radicals. We highly recommend extracts of grape seed, bilberry, and huckleberry; they're all available in capsule and tablet form.

Kidney and Bladder Tonic Formula

This recipe requires that you fill your own capsules, but the results are worth the work. Materials for doing so can be purchased at most larger health-food stores or mail-ordered from herb distributors listed in the Resource Directory. Purchase the herbs in powdered form.

Equal parts (one to two teaspoons) of the following:
Nettle leaf
Pipsissewa
Saw palmetto
Cranberry juice powder

and 1/2 part of
Juniper berry
Goldenrod

Grind the herb powders very fine in a coffee grinder or blender on high speed, in several pulses of no more than 20 seconds at a time (blending for longer may overheat the herbs). Place the powder into 00-size capsules. Take 2 to 4 capsules, 3 times daily, before meals. If making your own capsules isn't possible, you can make a light decoction of some or all of the herbs, adding a little licorice to make it more palatable. The licorice also has soothing and immune-enhancing properties of its own. This formula can be used for up to 1 month.

Acute Bladder-Infection Formula

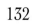

Use this formula to help heal an existing bladder infection.

1 ounce marshmallow root tincture
1 ounce echinacea tincture
1 ounce pipsissewa tincture
1/2 ounce usnea tincture
1/2 ounce uva ursi tincture
1/2 ounce Oregon grape root tincture
1/4 ounce myrrh tincture

Blend the tinctures together. Take 3 or 4 droppersful, 4 or 5 times a day, for up to 10 days. Take a break of 2 or 3 days, and then take another course if needed. Consult a physician and a qualified herbalist if your symptoms are persistent or severe.

Aromatherapy

The antiseptic essential oils found in juniper and tea tree can help fight bladder infection. Tea tree essential oil is a helpful topical antibiotic but don't take it internally without greatly diluting it; add no more than one drop of the pure essential oil per one ounce of tincture. Too much tea tree oil will irritate the urinary tract. A massage oil that contains tea tree oil, however, can be rubbed over the bladder area in addition to antibiotic or other herbal treatment.

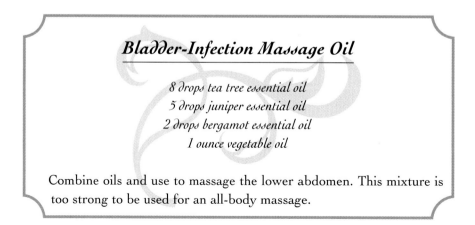

Bladder-Infection Massage Oil

8 drops tea tree essential oil
5 drops juniper essential oil
2 drops bergamot essential oil
1 ounce vegetable oil

Combine oils and use to massage the lower abdomen. This mixture is too strong to be used for an all-body massage.

CHAPTER 11

SEXUALLY TRANSMITTED DISEASES

For STDs, prevention is the best medicine. But when you have one, herbal therapies can be a powerful partner to medical solutions.

Sexually transmitted diseases (STDs) were once called venereal diseases after Venus, the Roman goddess of love. The viruses, bacteria, and other organisms that cause these diseases infect more than 12 million Americans each year. STDs also account for hundreds of thousands of deaths worldwide.

For centuries, syphilis and gonorrhea were the primary STDs. We became less concerned about these diseases when we learned fifty years ago that antibiotics would cure them. Ironically, the misuse of these powerful drugs has helped create antibiotic-resistant strains of these infections, and they are again on the rise. Meanwhile AIDS, or acquired immune-deficiency syndrome, infects 10 million people worldwide. About 75 percent of these infections occur by sexual transmission.

Unlike syphilis and AIDS, however, most STDs are not life-threatening. Some, however, such as chlamydia and genital warts, can lead to serious illnesses such as pelvic inflammatory disease and cervical cancer. Others, such as pubic lice, are merely annoying.

Diagnosing STDs

Women under the age of 25 are more likely than older women to contract a sexually transmitted disease, but STDs can infect anyone who engages in sexual activity. Younger women, however, often take fewer precautions during sex and have more contacts with more partners than others. Abstinence from sexual activity, though not popular, is the only sure way to prevent STDs; a completely

Echinacea

monogamous relationship between two healthy people is the next best, though not foolproof. Wearing a latex condom is somewhat protective, but this barrier can break, and a condom isn't 100-percent effective against such STDs as genital herpes. In addition, many STDs can exist—and be transmitted—without evincing symptoms in either party.

If you or your partner have had a number of sexual contacts, you are at greater risk for STDs. Many health authorities recommend getting a checkup every three months to six months. Only an annual gynecological exam is necessary if you maintain a long-term monogamous relationship.

During these checkups, you will be asked about your sexual contacts. A doctor will make a thorough pelvic examination, possibly including discharge samples from the vagina, urethra, or other sites, and will note inflammation, sores, or other abnormalities. If your tests are positive, your sexual partners may be notified, tested, and treated.

BACTERIAL STDs

Gonorrhea, chlamydia, and syphilis are among the bacterial STDs. If treated promptly, they can be completely eliminated from your body and cause no further problems. If left untreated, they can lead to severe ailments such as heart disease, blindness, or arthritis—even death.

Chlamydia

Nearly unknown a decade ago, chlamydia now accounts for four million new infections annually in the United States. Only recently have reliable tests for this infection been available. Chlamydia may produce no symptoms at all. When symptoms do appear, they usually include inflammation of the urethra and cervix, burning urination, excessive vaginal bleeding, fever, and abdominal pain, usually two or three weeks after infection. In up to 10 percent of cases, pelvic inflammatory disease (PID) occurs.

Untreated chlamydia causes 20 to 40 percent of female infertility and some tubal pregnancies. It can be passed to the baby during childbirth and cause pneumonia, eye infection, and blindness. Having chlamydia also increases a woman's risk of developing cervical dysplasia.

What a Doctor Will Do

The primary treatment is a one-week course of doxycycline, although it has side effects and drug interactions. Other antibiotics may also be prescribed.

Gonorrhea

Called "the clap" since the fourteenth century, gonorrhea is associated with the bacterium *Neisseria gonorrhoeae*. A woman is up to five times more likely to catch it from a man than vice versa. If a woman has one encounter with an infected male, her chance of infection is 90 percent. Most cases occur in people under age 20.

The incidence of gonorrhea decreased from the 1970s to the early 1990s, thanks to treatment with antibiotics. In 1991, over 600,000 cases were reported to disease-control centers in the United States, but in 1993, reported cases fell to 336,169. Cases of antibiotic-resistant gonorrhea are increasing, however.

The bacteria usually set up camp in the lower urinary tract or cervical canal but also can infect the mucous membranes of the throat or rectum. In women, the bacteria can migrate into the reproductive organs.

Symptoms can take from three days to three weeks to appear, but 80 percent of women and 10 percent of men with the infection develop no symptoms. Gonorrhea causes pain and burning with urination. When the pubic area is pressed, green or yellow-green pus may be discharged from the vagina or urethra. If the bacteria cause cervical inflammation, however, the only symptom may be increased vaginal discharge.

Men infected with gonorrhea typically feel burning and pain with urination and an increased urgency to urinate, sometimes with a yellowish-green discharge from the penis. If your partner develops these symptoms, you should be tested even if you show no signs of the disease.

What a Doctor Will Do

Testing for gonorrhea involves tissue cultures taken from the cervix, urethra, rectum, and throat; results usually are available in two or three days. If the test is positive, your sexual partner(s) should also be diagnosed and treated.

Doctors almost always prescribe antibiotics, especially in advanced cases, because these drugs work quickly. Be sure to know the side effects of the prescribed drug and ask about possible interactions with other drugs. We recommend coupling antibiotics with an immune-support program, including herbs such as echinacea, to help your body fight the illness.

Syphilis

Syphilis is associated with a tiny spiral organism, *Treponema pallidum*, called a spirochete. The organism is moderately transmissible by sexual intercourse; one exposure carries a 30-percent risk of infection. Since the development of antibiotics, syphilis has decreased. More recently, the incidence of syphilis has increased again because testing is no longer required to obtain a marriage license. More than 128,000 cases were reported in the United States in 1991, 45 percent of whom were women.

Syphilis is a three-stage disease spread by kissing; vaginal, anal and oral intercourse; and from mother to child during birth. In the first stage, ten to ninety days after exposure, a small, painless sore, called a chancre, with raised, even edges appears, usually wherever sexual contact occurred. The sore goes away in two to six weeks, but six weeks to six months later, the infected person feels general fatigue and malaise, often accompanied by swollen lymph nodes, sore throat, headaches, weight loss, and perhaps a painless rash over large parts of the body. Wart-like bumps appear on the perineum; these are called condyloma lata. After a few months, these symptoms disappear too, although they may reappear over the next year or so. This stage is followed by a latent period lasting up to ten years, during which no symptoms occur. In the third stage, serious, life-threatening damage to the heart, eyes, ears, and nervous system may occur.

What a Doctor Will Do

Diagnosis of syphilis is made with a blood test and examination of the fluid taken from a sore. Treatment consists of injections of benzathine penicillin; dosage and length of treatment depend on the stage of syphilis.

Viral STDs

Genital Warts

Warts are the most common viral STD, and the incidence is increasing worldwide. In the United States, about 50 million people are thought to be infected. Women under the age of 22 are more likely than others to be infected, and the incidence of infection declines after age 30. Because health workers are not required to report cases of genital warts, figures are uncertain.

Genital warts are small, flat or mushroom-shaped growths appearing singly or in clusters on the genitals of either sex. Usually painless, they are associated with certain types of human papilloma virus. Only 30 percent of those infected develop visible warts; 70 percent have subclinical infections in which no warts develop. Unfortunately, these subclinical infections are most often linked to cervical dysplasia. The disease may also enter a latent phase, residing in the body and remaining contagious without symptoms.

The virus is transmitted through the skin, usually during intercourse. Four weeks to nine months after exposure, blistery sores with a red base may appear on the labia first and then spread to other parts of the genital area, the anus, and buttocks. The infected area may become itchy. After their first appearance, the warts may stay the same, grow larger, or completely disappear. Even if the warts disappear, the virus remains in the body in a latent phase and reappear months or years later.

Risk factors for genital warts include multiple sex partners, cigarette smoking, and immune weakness. Infection with the viruses that cause genital warts is likely to be the most important risk factor for developing severe cervical dysplasia and cervical cancer. If you do test positive for a genital warts virus, be sure to get regular Pap smears and pelvic exams. The virus can remain latent for years and then trigger an abnormal Pap smear and cervical dysplasis.

What a Doctor Will Do

The genital warts viruses are hard to detect because they can't be cultured and no easy test for them exists. If exposure is suspected, a 3- to 5-percent acetic acid solution can be swabbed over the genital area, turning barely visible warts a noticeable white. A magnifying instrument called a colposcope helps identify very small lesions.

The treatment of genital warts is mostly symptomatic, because no treatment can remove the virus from the body. The warts themselves can be removed by freezing, surgery, laser or electric burning, or toxic chemicals, but they recur in up to 75 percent of cases. An effective vaccine may be several years away.

Because warts disappear spontaneously 20 to 30 percent of the time, you may wish to try a natural treatment program to support your immune system and discourage the virus. Whatever happens with the warts, be sure to have a Pap smear every six months to a year to check for cervical dysplasia.

> ## HERPES, WARTS, AND PAP SMEARS
>
> Herpes infections are not life-threatening, but they do increase the risk of developing cervical dysplasia and cervical cancer, especially in women who also are infected with the genital warts virus. If you have both genital herpes and genital warts, you should have a Pap test every six months to a year.

Genital Herpes

Genital herpes is a common STD from the herpes family of viruses; other members cause chickenpox and cold sores. Two common herpes viruses infect humans, HSV1 and HSV2. Both viruses can affect the genital areas, but usually HSV1 is associated with blisters of the mouth and tongue while HSV2 is associated with lesions of the genitals. There is no known cure or vaccine for herpes after the initial infection. The virus travels up nerves to nerve cells along the spine, where it lies dormant until a stressor reactivates it.

Because up to 70 percent of those infected with genital herpes display no symptoms, the virus spreads easily between sexual partners. Some mistakenly believe that the virus can be transmitted only when sores can be seen. Wrong: genital herpes is so insidious and so widespread that an estimated 200,000 people are newly infected each year in the United States alone. By age 30, 20 percent of white women carry the virus.

Infected women typically develop sores of the vulva, cervix, or anus. They often feel tingling or itching before the outbreak. The first episode, almost always the most severe and painful, can last up to two weeks. Swollen lymph nodes, sore muscles, and headaches usually accompany the sores. Outbreaks usually last four or five days; blisters heal in one to three weeks. There is no immunity to genital herpes.

Factors that can trigger an outbreak of latent HSV2 include stress, weakened immunity, diet, surgery, skin rashes, menstruation, hormonal fluctuations, or prolonged sexual activity. Exposure to sunlight, especially when mouth lesions are involved, also can bring on outbreaks. These episodes, at least, are easily prevented by using sunscreen.

What a Doctor Will Do

It's easiest to diagnose potential herpes when sores are obvious. A Pap smear, a Tzanck smear, or cell cultures can be used. Some labs can culture the fluid from a sore in about a week. A blood test that detects genital herpes antibodies is available but not reliable.

The antiviral drug Acyclovir (Zovirax) is commonly prescribed in both pill and ointment form, especially for the initial outbreak. Most effective when taken at the first sign of outbreak, Acyclovir speeds healing of blisters and may reduce other symptoms without severe side effects. The safety of the drug during pregnancy is unproven. Pain relievers, both oral and topical, are also prescribed.

HIV and AIDS

More than 46,000 women in the United States and more than 600,000 worldwide have AIDS. In fact, AIDS is the leading cause of death worldwide for ages men and women 25 to 44, and the fourth most common cause of death in the United States. Worldwide, about 75 percent of AIDS cases result from sexual intercourse, and 80 percent of these are heterosexually transmitted. Some researchers believe that eventually the rate of heterosexual transmission of AIDS will exceed that of homosexual transmission in the United States.

We can't possibly discuss all aspects of HIV and AIDS here—entire books have been written about it—so we will include basic nutritional and herbal programs for supporting the immune system and managing other symptoms associated with the disease. A number of excellent books about HIV/AIDS exist, many with a natural-healing orientation.

For women, HIV infection can increase the likelihood of developing severe and recurrent forms of other STDs. A Pap smear with colposcopic exam every six months is a wise precaution. If you experience unexplained symptoms such as chronic fatigue, generalized lymph-node swelling, diarrhea, persistent infections, and especially yeast infections in the throat (thrush) or vagina, consult your physician or get a test for HIV at a state or local clinic.

AIDS testing is available through state, county, and city health clinics and from some private doctors. It is also sometimes available from non-profit women's clinics. The test, called ELISA, detects antibodies produced by the body in response to the virus. However, these antibodies may not develop for two to six months after exposure, so repeated tests during that time may be required. The most important reason for regular testing is to prevent spreading the virus to others.

What a Doctor Will Do

Three major drug treatments have developed over the last few years to treat AIDS, the disease associated with HIV.

- Reverse transcriptase drugs block the virus from reproducing itself. These include AZT (Zidovudine).
- The new protease inhibitors are especially effective when combined with reverse transcriptase inhibitors.
- Antibiotics such as Septra (trimethoprim-sulfamethoxazole) kill opportunistic, infectious pathogens such as *Pneumocystis carinii*, which causes the notorious "AIDS pneumonia."

Although these drugs have slowed the death rate from AIDS, they do not work for everyone. Side effects can be debilitating, and the virus sometimes becomes resistant.

OTHER STDS AND COMPLICATIONS

Pelvic Inflammatory Disease (PID)

Pelvic inflammatory disease results when a pathogen—the microbes that cause gonorrhea or chlamydia, for example—invades the reproductive organs: the uterus, ovaries, or fallopian tubes. The symptoms of PID include fever, chills, nausea, pain during urination and intercourse, heavy menstrual flow with severe cramps, increasing lower abdominal pain, and sometimes vaginal bleeding. Some women have no symptoms until the disease is advanced. Appendicitis, tubal pregnancy, endometriosis, miscarriage or abortion complications, and other conditions produce symptoms very similar to those of PID, so prompt investigation is important.

Scar tissue resulting from PID is the primary cause of infertility and tubal pregnancies in North American women, but prompt treatment reduces the risk of these and other complications. The National Institute of Child Health and Human Development reports that women who smoke double their risk of developing PID.

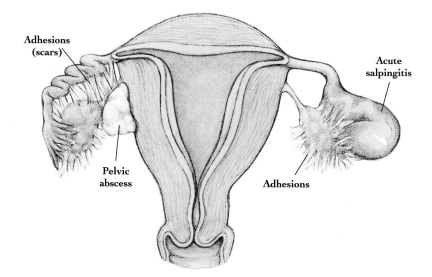

Pelvic inflammatory disease and possible complications

What a Doctor Will Do

Diagnostic measures for PID often include blood work, a culture, and/or a laparoscopy. PID can be treated with antibiotics such as cefozxitin, cefotetan, and doxycycline, given intravenously if necessary, and bed rest. Women with acute PID are usually hospitalized. Severe cases can require hysterectomy.

Pubic Lice

Also known as "crabs," these small lice are highly transmissible by genital-to-genital contact and infected clothing, sheets, toilet seats, and blankets. They inhabit the hairy areas of the body, where they feed on blood. The eggs, called nits, are found attached to the bases of individual hairs. Two to four weeks after infection, intense itching and perhaps a red rash develop in the affected area. Mild fever, irritability, and fatigue may also develop.

What a Doctor Will Do

Diagnosis is easy because the lice are clearly visible under a magnifying glass. The doctor will prescribe an insecticide shampoo containing Lindane, such as Kwell, or a 1-percent permethrin cream rinse, which is preferable. It is normal to feel itchy for a few days after the lice are killed. The least noxious treatment may be an over-the-counter preparation containing a pyrethrin derivative with piperonyl butoxide (Rid). This is applied for ten minutes and then removed with soap and water. Some women are allergic to these chemical treatments, so be careful.

NATURAL HEALING FOR STDs

Healthy Habits

Because many STDs can be asymptomatic—in other words, you or your partner can have them, and transmit them, while showing no signs—prevention is probably the healthiest habit you can practice. Barrier contraceptives such as condoms help but are not 100-percent effective, even against AIDS. If you are sexually active and not in a monogamous relationship, get frequent, regular checkups. If you are in a monogamous relationship and show symptoms of an STD, get a diagnosis promptly.

Dietary Changes

If you contract an STD and are being treated with antibiotics, help your body adjust to these powerful drugs by eliminating as much sugar from your diet as you can. Take a probiotic supplement to help replenish the friendly bacteria that the antibiotics kill. For more about probiotics, see the Vaginal Infections chapter.

Herbal Healing

In most STD cases, echinacea can help. You may want to embark on a complete program of immune boosters such as echinacea and liver-support herbs such as milk thistle as outlined in the chapter on vaginal infections, especially if your STD is bacterial.

If it is viral, a number of herbs have proven virus-inhibiting effects. The most widely used include garlic and St. John's wort. Here are dosages for common anti-viral herbs.

- Garlic: Two to four capsules daily; can be used for long periods.
- St. John's wort: Four droppersful of liquid extract, morning and evening, every other day.
- Osha: Three droppersful of the liquid extract twice daily.
- Isatis: Two of the three droppersful of tincture, two to three times daily.
- Licorice: Two to three cups of decoction daily, for up to two weeks.
- Shiitake: Two to four capsules or tablets of the powdered extract, twice daily.

External Applications

For irritation, redness, and itching of the vulva, apply a cream or a light salve containing such soothing herbs as aloe vera, calendula, chamomile, or plantain leaf. You can add one part aloe vera gel to one part calendula or chamomile cream yourself. Apply to irritated membranes morning and evening or as needed. Avoid creams that contain perfumes or essential oils that might irritate sensitive mucous membranes.

Specific Remedies: Genital Herpes

Dietary adjustments. Many succeed in managing genital herpes by limiting intake of foods containing arginine while increasing those with lysine. Arginine-rich foods to be avoided include chocolate, peanuts and peanut butter, walnuts, hazelnuts, and Brazil nuts. Foods high in lysine are turkey, chicken, fish, cottage cheese, ricotta cheese, and wheat germ.

Supplements. One respected practitioner with extensive clinical experience recommends that genital herpes sufferers take 3 grams of lysine daily for three months, then 1 gram daily afterwards to prevent outbreaks. Vitamin E supplements (400 to 800 IU daily) may be beneficial; you can also apply vitamin E oil topically to reduce pain and accelerate healing. Taking 600 mg or more of vitamin C may reduce outbreak length and inhibit lesion formation.

Zinc may reduce the severity or length of genital herpes outbreaks. Zinc is a powerful, broad-spectrum antiviral and antioxidant that can enhance certain immune functions. Try zinc when you first notice tingling or other signs of outbreak, and continue for a few days after the acute phase passes. Then cut back to normal zinc levels and continue your usual multivitamin and mineral supplements.

Topical remedies. A recent patent was filed for using black tea for herpes to reduce pain and inflammation, probably in part because it contains astringent tannins. Of course, you can also make a simple home treatment: Simply steep a black tea bag for a few minutes in just enough boiling water to cover. Let the bag cool and apply directly to the herpes lesion.

Herpes/Immune-System Tincture

1/2 teaspoon echinacea tincture
1/2 teaspoon St. John's wort tincture
1/2 teaspoon Chinese bupleurum tincture
1/2 teaspoon licorice root tincture
1/2 teaspoon barberry tincture

Combine the tinctures. Take one dropperful of the tincture four to six times daily.

Topical Herpes Treatment

If the alcohol of the tinctures stings too much when you use this treatment, substitute glycerites or diluted infused oils of the same herbs.

1/2 teaspoon St. John's wort tincture
1/2 teaspoon licorice root tincture
5 drops tea tree essential oil
3 drops myrrh essential oil

Combine all ingredients. Shake well before applying. Apply not more than two to three times a day directly on the herpes lesion.

Another promising treatment for reducing herpes outbreaks is lemon balm, applied topically or taken as a tea. Lemon-balm ointments and creams are widely available and should be applied to the outbreak area or to the lesions; follow the directions on the package. Drinking a tea of fresh or dried lemon balm is a pleasant, lemony way to reduce symptoms. Use the tea daily when you feel an outbreak coming on, or simply as a periodic preventative.

Zinc creams treat external sores; a study of 158 volunteers at the Chiang Mai University, Thailand, found that a zinc monoglycerolate preparation penetrates the skin and inhibits viral replication while speeding the healing of blisters. Topical applications of zinc sulfate ointment can reduce pain, length of outbreak, and recurrence of infection.

Vitamin E oil, aloe vera gel, or plantain juice or cream can be applied directly to the lesions to encourage healing and reduce scarring. We have found St. John's wort tincture or oil effective for reducing the pain and burning of the sores when applied twice daily.

In China, a strong infusion of the herb *Yu xing cao* is used as a compress for reducing the pain of herpes sores and assisting healing. We recommend making a tea by simmering a tablespoon of herb in a cup of water for ten minutes; remove from heat and let stand for 30 to 45 minutes. Soak a sterile cotton pad in the tea and tape over the sores. Change two or three times daily.

Aromatherapy for Herpes

Essential oils that may help battle the herpes virus are bergamot, tea tree, lavender, and lemon balm. They also seem to noticeably reduce the discomfort, extent, and duration of the outbreak. Herbalist Jane Bothwell highly recommends essential oil of myrrh. We find that it works at least as well, if not better, than the other essential oils, but it is expensive. If you use bergamot, make sure to get bergaptene-free essential oil, since this constituent can cause skin reactions in sunlight.

Specific Remedies: Genital Warts

Aromatherapy offers natural alternatives to treating genital warts. The essential oils of tea tree and thuja eliminate genital warts in some women. Since these oils are quite potent—and they need to be to destroy warts—use them carefully. Dilute the essential oil in an equal part of castor oil, then apply only to the wart. This preparation can burn sensitive skin areas, so first protect the skin around the wart with salve, leaving only the wart exposed. If you do not see results in a week or so,

> ## *Genital Wart Oil*
>
> *1/2 teaspoon castor oil*
> *1/4 teaspoon thuja essential oil*
> *1/4 teaspoon tea tree essential oil*
> *800 units vitamin E oil (2 opened capsules)*
>
> Combine ingredients. Carefully apply the mixture only to the wart with a cotton swab, two to four times daily.

consult a doctor. If your warts are inside the vagina or on the cervix, a naturopathic doctor can apply the above preparation or a similar one.

Specific Remedies: Syphilis

Syphilis is a progressive disease that requires treatment with an antibiotic such as penicillin. Natural treatments to help the antibiotics do their job, and help your body recover from them, include immune toners and herbs to support the digestion.

To ease the pain of sores, try applying aloe vera gel, plantain or comfrey leaf juice, or tea compresses.

Traditional Chinese Medicine hospitals use a formula of Chinese sarsaparilla along with Japanese honeysuckle flowers, licorice root, Chinese dittany root, purslane, and dandelion root to treat syphilis. These herbs can be found in Chinese herb shops or purchased from many acupuncturists.

Specific Remedies: Pubic Lice

Some cases of lice respond to a 10-percent sulfur cream or ointment, available at some pharmacies. Add 10 drops of eucalyptus or tea tree essential oil per ounce to cut the sulfur smell and increase effectiveness. Apply the ointment over the affected area before bedtime for three consecutive nights, washing it off each morning. If you can't find the sulfur ointment, you can make your own by melting calendula salve in a double boiler or saucepan under low heat and mixing in 10-percent flowers of sulfur, available from pharmacies. Nit combs, available from drug stores, remove the eggs without chemicals.

Make sure to thoroughly wash all sheets, towels, and clothing every day that you apply the salve.

Specific Remedies: PID

Herbs and diet alone rarely heal PID. A course of antibiotics plus an herbal antibiotic support program, as described in the previous chapter, often yield the best results. Prevention is essential to avoiding PID. If a vaginal infection begins, treat it promptly and keep it from recurring with a low-sugar diet and other healthy strategies.

Immune-stimulation therapy is especially important in combating acute PID. Take echinacea tincture (two or three droppersful, four times daily), eat lots of chlorophyll-rich foods, and drink fresh juices. Six to eight ounces of parsley or wheat-grass juice can be taken two or three times daily. Liquids, powders, capsules, or tablets containing spirulina and/or barley grass may also help.

A twice-daily sitz bath can help relieve intense pain in cases of PID. Castor-oil packs twice daily are also recommended. Both foot reflexology and visualization may be beneficial as well.

Specific Remedies: HIV/AIDS

The best healing strategy for HIV/AIDS sufferers is one aimed at strengthening the immune system, hormones, nervous system, and overall vitality. Herbal therapy can play a significant role whether it is used with or without drugs.

Immune support and digestive vitality support are essential, because the HIV virus often severely weakens these systems. Herbs that inhibit viral growth are essential. We strongly recommend acupuncture, massage, and counseling to help release stress, tension, and negative emotions. The diet should be highly nutritious, easy to assimilate, and free of processed foods, refined sugar products, stimulants, and alcohol. Use superfoods such as spirulina and nettle-leaf tea or extract to support vital energy production and the function of enzyme systems.

Two antiviral herbs to try in HIV/AIDS cases include St. John's wort and bitter melon. St. John's wort is available in many health food stores and mainstream pharmacies. Take 900 mg per day in two doses for three days, then stop for one day; repeat for up to nine months or longer as needed. Or take 3/4 teaspoon of a tincture twice daily for the same amount of time. The juice or powder of bitter melon, taken orally, may be useful; it is available in many Chinese food stores.

CHAPTER 12

CERVICAL DYSPLASIA

"Your Pap test shows cervical dysplasia." Every year, thousands of women hear their doctors say these words, and many are stricken with fear. What does "cervical dysplasia" mean? Is it cancer? What happens next?

Cervical dysplasia means that abnormal cells exist on the cervix, the slender entrance to the uterus. The condition is classified as mild, moderate, or severe. Dysplasia is *not* cancer, but it can be a precursor of cervical cancer, a common cancer among women. The more advanced the dysplasia, the more likely it is to become cancerous. What happens next depends on the degree of the condition, but careful monitoring of even mild cervical dysplasia is essential.

Ignored, some cervical dysplasia can become cancerous, first involving only the surface cells of the cervix, then deeper cells; it can spread to the upper vagina and uterus. Full-blown cancer can invade other organs and enter the lymphatic system, by which it can travel and establish itself throughout the body. For women whose cancer becomes this widespread, the five-year survival rate is only about 40 percent.

Yet most women diagnosed with cervical dysplasia do not develop cancer. Instead, they recover fully. About one-third of mild cases spontaneously regress. However, after a first abnormal Pap test, doctors often will examine cervical tissue more closely to evaluate the extent of the abnormality. Results can range from slight inflammation to a cancerous or precancerous condition.

For some women, the abnormalities revealed by a Pap test heal without treatment. For others, the early warnings provided by annual Pap tests and the array of effective herbal and medical treatments available offer chances to defeat cervical dysplasia before it becomes cancer.

Burdock

Nearly every woman with cervical dysplasia may choose from several helpful options. She also has time to consider these options and make a well-considered, informed decision. It usually takes ten or more years for cancer to develop from mild dysplasia, according to the National Cancer Institute, although those caused by aggressive forms of the human papilloma virus can progress rapidly.

Most likely, your doctor will wait a month or more, then repeat your Pap test to be sure of the results. In the meantime, you can develop a natural health program that includes exercise and a healthy diet with sufficient nutrients and no toxins. We know from the experience of many women that this commitment to healing makes a big difference.

THE STATISTICS

Just how common is cervical dysplasia? And what are a woman's chances that it will become cancer? The United States does not keep statistics on this condition, making it impossible to ascertain how many mild dysplasias result in cervical cancer, although the figure is estimated at 15 percent. Some studies have attempted to determine these statistics in other populations, however. When we looked for research that tried to determine the incidence of cervical dysplasia and probable outcomes, the numbers varied widely.

A New Zealand study spanning 1980 through 1986 examined the health of 9,302 women from the general population. Of these, 4.3 percent had cervical dysplasia or cancer.

In two studies conducted in India, researchers examined 4,338 and 66,736 women; the smaller study reported dysplasia in 4.6 percent of subjects, while the larger found it in only 1.4 percent.

Contrast these figures with a study of European women: Of 870 women age 20 or younger, 11 percent had dysplasia. Typically, the problem occurs most often among women ages 33 to 38.

While testing for dysplasia is not always accurate and these studies face other limitations, the following conclusions can be made.

The incidence of cervical dysplasia in North America is unknown. Of 870 European women age 20 or younger, 11 percent had the condition. In a much larger study of more than 66,000 Indian women, only 1.4 percent had dysplasia.

- Some who received no treatment healed completely.

- Between 11 and 62 percent of untreated women had improved when examined several months to a few years later.

- Between 22 and 64 percent of untreated women were worse when examined several months to a few years later.

- About 25 percent advanced to severe dysplasia.

- About 16 percent developed cervical cancer.

Many factors affect the development of any cancer: the patient's general health, strength of the immune system, diet, availability of medical care, and more. In addition, different medical centers can define dysplasia differently. So it is not surprising to find a wide range of outcomes.

The severity of a woman's dysplasia strongly influences her chances of developing cervical cancer. Mild cases are more likely to heal than moderate and severe ones; these are more likely to progress to cervical cancer. Some physicians see cervical dysplasia as the first sign of cervical cancer, but the progression is far from inevitable.

When a woman has mild dysplasia and follow-up tests do not indicate a cancerous condition, watchful waiting—frequent Pap tests but no rush to treatment—may be the best course. More advanced conditions require more careful monitoring.

WHY ME? THE RISK FACTORS

Women can powerfully influence their risk for developing cervical dysplasia by practicing safe sex, avoiding cigarette smoking, and having regular Pap tests. While other factors certainly affect the development of the problem, many cases of cervical dysplasia can be avoided by eliminating these risk factors alone.

Sexually Transmitted Diseases

While scientists have long suspected that cancer is triggered or perhaps even caused by unknown infectious agents, the theory has been hard to prove. Recent research into cervical dysplasia and cervical cancer, however, has shown strikingly high correlations between these conditions and sexually transmitted viruses.

A large body of research shows that cervical dysplasia is strongly encouraged by some strains of the human papilloma virus. Scientists have identified some fifty varieties of this virus. Some cause common warts of the hands and feet, while others result in lesions of the mucous membranes in the mouth, genitals, and anal cavity. Some types are strongly associated with cervical cancer.

Infection with one of the viruses that causes genital warts often precedes cervical dysplasia. In one study, researchers found that women with cervical dysplasia are six times more likely to be infected with genital wart viruses than other women. Researchers also have found that the amount of the virus concentrated in tissues and active in the body is a good predictor of whether the body will heal the dysplasia on its own. High tissue levels of the virus are associated with a poorer outcome, especially if the virus is an aggressive type.

Human papilloma virus is a sexually transmitted disease. Unfortunately, it can be asymptomatic—meaning that it shows no symptoms. In our practices, we encounter many men and some women who don't know that that the virus is contagious and can be passed to sexual partners. Certainly many are unaware that the virus is strongly associated with cervical dysplasia and possibly cancer.

Dysplasia is also promoted by the virus that causes genital herpes, *Herpes simplex* type II. A study of 112 women who had either cervical dysplasia or cervical cancer turned up a 78-percent rate of genital herpes infection; in the control group of 42 women, the incidence of genital herpes was only about 2 percent. And in the 55 women with cervical cancer, 50 women tested positive for the virus.

The same study also examined the possible effects on cervical dysplasia and cancer when several viruses are present. It found that when a woman has both genital warts and genital herpes, the chance of her developing cervical dysplasia and eventually cancer increases. In addition, those infected with the viruses had more severe conditions.

Infection with the human immunodeficiency virus—HIV, the virus associated with AIDS—also correlates highly with cervical dysplasia. Researchers found in 1993 that not only were HIV-positive women more likely than others to have cervical problems, but that the progres-

RISK FACTORS FOR CERVICAL DYSPLASIA

Infection with one of the human papilloma viruses that causes genital warts

Infection with *Herpes simplex* II, which causes genital herpes

Infection with (HIV), the virus associated with AIDS

Infection with hepatitis B or C virus

Male sex partner has genital warts, herpes, HIV, or contact with another partner who carries such infections

Many sexual partners, especially during the teenage years

First sexual intercourse at a young age

Smoking more than twenty cigarettes a day

Taking birth control pills for more than ten years

Taking immunosuppressive drugs following organ transplant

Deficiency in folic acid, vitamin A, and/or beta-carotene

Many pregnancies

sion of their condition could be more rapid and its severity intensified. Women who carry the HIV virus are more likely than others to be infected with genital herpes and warts.

The connection between the usual transmission mode of these diseases and cervical dysplasia may explain why lesbian women have a relatively low risk of dysplasia. Cervical dysplasia occurs in only about 3 percent of lesbian women. When these women do have an increased risk, it is associated with past heterosexual contacts or factors unrelated to sexuality, such as smoking.

Cigarettes and cervical dysplasia

Not all risk factors for cervical dysplasia are related to sexual behavior. Smoking cigarettes, long-term use of estrogen-based birth-control pills, and folic acid deficiency also increase your risk. Several of these conditions can combine with other risk factors to raise the possibility of abnormal cell growth.

Dysplasia is two to three times more likely to occur in women who smoke cigarettes than in those who don't. It is also more often severe in smokers. In fact, nicotine, a toxin found in cigarette smoke, shows up in the cervical secretions of women who smoke and in smaller amounts in those who are exposed to passive smoke. One study shows that the chance of having cervical dysplasia steadily increases along with the number of cigarettes a woman smokes.

Other risk factors

Many women with cervical dysplasia have a deficiency in the nutrient folic acid, a part of the B-vitamin complex that is sometimes also called folate. Among women who take birth-control pills or drink heavily, the nutrient also tends to be low. Some doctors automatically suspect a folic acid deficiency when tests show abnormal cervical cells. One recent study shows that those who use oral contraceptives for four years or less increase their risk by only a few percentage points, but another finds notably increased risk among those who use the pills for ten years or more, although the number of sexual partners and smoking remain the most important risk factors for cervical dysplasia in the study.

Excessive estrogen, whether synthetic or produced by the body, can also increase the chance of cervical dysplasia or cancer. Women exposed prenatally to a synthetic estrogen called DES (diethylstilbestrol) are at special risk of cervical dysplasia and vaginal cancer. The drug was prescribed to expectant mothers from the 1940s through the 1960s to prevent miscarriage. Only when the daughters of these mothers reached maturity did it become clear that the daughters developed cervical dysplasia and cancers of the reproductive system at higher rates than the general population; the drug is now forbidden during pregnancy. Careful monitoring is required for DES daughters.

In fact, we believe that anything that lowers general immune ability probably contributes to cervical dysplasia and cancer. For instance, immune-suppressing drugs that must be taken following an organ transplant raise the risk of dysplasia, as do stress and ongoing problems with cervical inflammation. A weak immune system is ill-prepared to fight invasive disease. In addition to other benefits, improving the overall health of your reproductive organs and immune system will reduce your risk of many reproductive disorders.

> *Women who smoke are two to three times more likely to develop cervical dysplasia, and it is more often severe.*

WHAT A DOCTOR WILL DO

The Pap Test: A Good Insurance Policy

The Pap test, named after the American medical researcher George N. Papanicolaou, has been used for early detection and prevention of cervical cancer since the 1950s. According to a panel of experts commissioned by the National Institute of Health in 1996, Pap smear screening remains the best available method of reducing the incidence and mortality of invasive cervical cancer.

Thanks to this test, cases of cervical cancer have steadily declined by as much as 50 percent since 1958, when its use became commonplace. Likewise, deaths from cervical cancer have dropped by up to 70 percent in communities where Pap smears and another common test, colposcopy, or vaginal examination with a small scope, are used often. Recent figures show that half the women diagnosed with cervical cancer have never had a Pap smear. Discontinuing regular Pap smears after the childbearing years is a bad idea; 20 percent of cervical cancer patients are elderly.

How Often Should You Be Tested?

How often to have a Pap smear is somewhat controversial. One study shows that having the test done every three years offers as much protection as annual tests.

The American Cancer Society recommends that women age 18 and older and all sexually active women have annual Pap tests until they have had four or more sequential negative tests. After that, less frequent screenings at three-year intervals are sufficient for women who are not at high risk.

The American College of Obstetrics and Gynecology, however, recommends annual Pap tests for most women, because it can be difficult to determine high-risk groups. Older women who are in a stable, monogamous relationship can be screened less frequently.

We recommend that women should continue Pap testing beyond the age of childbearing, and lesbian women should get Pap smears as often as heterosexual women. Above all, don't miss your regular Pap smears if you smoke, have had multiple sex partners, if your overall health is poor, or if your mother took DES before you were born. If you have a good diet and health habits, you have no specific risk factors, and your most recent test was normal, a Pap test every three years is probably all you need.

What the Test Involves

If you are scheduled for a Pap test, you can maximize its accuracy. Avoid douching or using a tampon for three days prior to your exam. Don't have intercourse for at least twenty-four hours, and preferably forty-eight hours, beforehand. Many doctors request that you schedule an appointment at least a week after your menstrual period is finished. In addition, if you've had a vaginal infection, wait at least a week before the Pap smear.

To take a Pap smear, the doctor inserts a swab, small spatula, or stiff brush into the end of the cervical canal and rotates it to pick up a sampling of the cells. Samples may also be taken from outside the cervix and the vagina wall. These are smeared onto a slide and examined under a microscope to check for abnormalities. If mild dysplasia is reported from the Pap test, the doctor will often request another test to confirm or rule out the diagnosis.

A colposcopic exam is often the next test ordered when a Pap smear detects abnormal cells. To help the physician see abnormal areas,

HOW OFTEN DO I NEED A PAP TEST?

The National Cancer Institute recommends the following:

Begin Pap smears when you become sexually active or reach age 18.

Screen regularly; discuss the frequency of your exams with your doctor.

Risk factors such as intercourse prior to age 18, unprotected sex with multiple partners, sexually transmitted diseases, and smoking increase the need for screening.

Hysterectomy, the removal of the uterus and cervix, does not always rule out the need for continued Pap tests. Consult your doctor about whether you need further tests.

a 3-percent acetic acid solution is swabbed on the cervix; abnormal areas turn white and opaque and are readily identified. Then a colposcope, a lighted microscope, is positioned outside the vagina. The doctor using it can detect subtle changes in cervical cells as well as other irregularities or problems.

Remember, It's Only a Test

Remember that a Pap test is only a screening procedure and not accurate enough to diagnose dysplasia. It is nonetheless a good way to monitor the health of the cervix and help you determine when you should take further action.

Improved techniques in taking cell samples and better quality standards in the laboratories where the samples are read have made Pap smears more accurate, but false negatives still crop up in about 20 percent of the tests. This means that abnormal cells are sometimes not detected. False positives are also possible, so if a Pap test detects abnormal cells, it is important to repeat the test or have a colposcopic examination before you undergo more invasive testing. If you have had a positive Pap test, consider requesting a repeat test if your doctor has not recommended it.

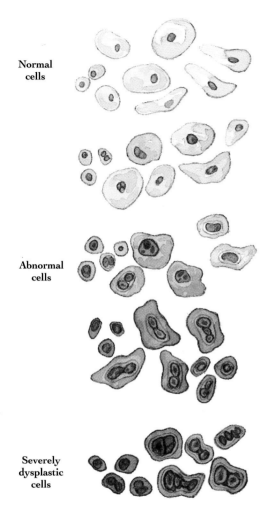

Normal cells

Abnormal cells

Severely dysplastic cells

Cervical cells showing increasingly serious dysplasia

What the Results Mean

Normal cervical cells are a type called squamous epithelial cells. "Squamous" is derived from the Latin word *squama*, meaning scale. In the cervix, stacks of these flat cells make up the epithelium, or outer layer. These terms—squamous and epithelial—recur in Pap-test reports that describe cellular and tissue abnormalities.

The accuracy of a Pap test depends upon several factors, including a proper sampling of the epithelial cells of the cervix, the quality of the staining of the cells, and the accuracy of the laboratory analysis. Below are some of the cell conditions that a Pap test and colposcopic exam may indicate, along with how your doctor may treat them.

- **Findings essentially normal.** This means that no abnormalities have been found to indicate dysplasia or cancer of the cervix. This is the most frequent result of a Pap test.

- **Inadequate sample.** Not enough cells were collected to make a determination. You should request a repeat test, even if your doctor disagrees.

- **Abnormalities that indicate infections.** Further testing is advised and may include microscopic examination of vaginal fluid and cultures to detect viral or bacterial infections.

- **Squamous cell abnormalities of undetermined significance.** Changes in epithelial cells are evident, but they are not clearly dysplasia. Your doctor may order repeat Pap smears or remove more cells and examine them under a microscope to identify abnormalities.

- **A low-grade squamous intraepithelial lesion.** This encompasses mild dysplasia and means the cells look abnormal. You can watch and wait, scheduling another test now or in three to six months, especially if you are in good health, have no risk factors associated with cervical dysplasia, and follow or plan to develop a natural health program. If you do have an increased risk—smoking, for example—a colposcopic examination can provide more precise information. This test is no more invasive than a regular pelvic exam.

- **A high-grade squamous intraepithelial lesion.** This category includes moderate and severe dysplasia as well as cancer *in situ* (in place). Moderate dysplasia indicates elevated numbers of distorted epithelial cells. In severe dysplasia, abnormal cells extend through two-thirds of the epithelium. When severe dysplasia is the diagnosis, colposcopy and biopsy of the affected tissue will almost certainly be recommended.

- **Carcinoma (or cancer) *in situ*.** In this condition, abnormal cells exist throughout the thickness of the epithelium, but they have not penetrated the membrane below. The carcinoma is almost always surgically removed; biopsy confirms the diagnosis. Additional tests such as X-ray, computed tomography, or magnetic resonance imaging will determine whether the cancer is localized or has spread to other areas of the body.

- **Invasive carcinoma.** Abnormal cells have penetrated the membrane lining and can spread to adjacent organs or the lymphatic system. A biopsy is necessary to determine whether the cancerous cells remain localized. The doctor will most often recommend removing the cancerous cells by conventional or laser surgery or other methods. Surgery may be followed by radiation therapy and chemotherapy.

Medical Treatment

To make informed decisions about the treatment of cervical dysplasia or cervical cancer, it's helpful to gain an understanding of the cells involved. Both cervical and epithelial cells can be involved in dysplasia.

The portion of the cervix located at the top of the vagina is covered by squamous epithelial cells; the cervical canal is lined with a single layer of columnar cells that secrete mucus. The doughnut-shaped border between these two types of cells, typically located around the opening of the cervix, is called the transformation zone. The transformation zone constantly shifts its position as women age and may even move inside the cervical canal.

Cells in this zone are very sensitive to changes within the vagina. They may respond to stimuli such as pH, toxins produced by the vagina's microflora or circulating in the bloodstream, substances in a sex partner's semen, douches, contraceptive foams, infections such as genital herpes or warts, or an IUD. Cervical dysplasia or cancer typically begins in this zone.

KNOW YOUR DIAGNOSTIC OPTIONS

Sometimes a physician recommends removing areas of abnormal cells during a colposcopy exam. Both curettage (scraping) and cone biopsy can be used. While this "one-step" combination of exam and cell gathering may save insurance companies money, the cell removal may not be essential.

According to some researchers, mild dysplasia does not warrant one-step treatment. In a study of simultaneous colposcopy and curettage, only 3 of 203 patients who underwent the procedure had dysplasia. The researchers concluded that routine curettage during the initial colposcopic examination added expense and caused significant patient discomfort, but yielded little additional information.

Curettage or cone biopsies may be more appropriate for women past menopause because the transformation area where dysplasia usually begins has often moved into the cervical canal. In these cases, the areas of abnormal cells can be partially or completely hidden, so the extra procedure may be justified.

When considering a cone biopsy, make a careful choice; it can cause internal scarring. Take time to gather information, seek the support of friends, and get a second opinion before undergoing any surgical procedure.

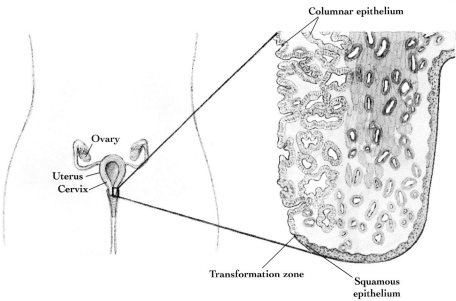

The cervix and transformation zone

Physicians generally suggest treating dysplasia by burning, freezing, or removing the problem cells with a laser, electric current, or surgery. Each treatment has special circumstances when it is most applicable.

Cryosurgery and Laser Surgery

Destroying abnormal cells by freezing (cryosurgery) or a laser is common. However, these techniques leave no abnormal cells behind for further diagnosis, so they are used only when:

• The transformation zone and any lesions are completely visible.

• Dysplasia areas do not extend into the cervical canal.

• Cancerous cells, or are not present.

When these conditions are met, cryosurgery is the most cost-effective method of treating dysplasia, since it can be performed in the office without anesthesia. If cancer is ruled out by colposcopy, the success rate of cryosurgery is about 92 percent. The cervix heals in one to two months. Infection is rare, and the procedure does not affect fertility. One drawback is that when the transformation zone grows back, it is more likely to migrate into the cervical canal. In about half the patients, it can no longer be fully seen for later examinations. Another drawback is ten to fourteen days of profuse, watery vaginal discharge.

In laser surgery, a carbon dioxide laser beam vaporizes the transformation zone along with any abnormal cells. Laser treatment is more costly than freezing and requires more expertise to perform, but it is more precise and requires a somewhat shorter recovery time. Its main drawback is that it is more painful than freezing and requires a local, or in some cases, general anesthesia. When the transformation zone grows back after laser treatment, it migrates to the cervical canal in only 15 percent of patients.

Cone Biopsy, Loop Electroexcision, and Hysterectomy

When the areas of abnormal cells are not clearly limited, doctors will usually choose conventional surgery. The removed tissue can be closely examined; if its edges are completely free of abnormal cells, treatment is complete. If abnormal cells exist at the edge of the sample, doctors will likely recommend further tissue removal.

A cone biopsy involves removing a cone-shaped section of the cervix, including the entire transformation zone, for examination under a microscope. The procedure allows a highly accurate diagnosis but can cause scarring of the cervix. The traditional method uses a scalpel. Local or general anesthesia is required, and bleeding frequently occurs.

The loop electroexcision procedure (called LEEP) has several advantages over cone biopsy because, instead of a scalpel, the procedure employs a small, electrically charged wire loop to remove abnormal cervical tissue. It coagulates blood at the same time, greatly reducing bleeding, and is inexpensive and easy to perform. In follow-up studies, women experience less discomfort and fewer complications, such as bleeding, than with cone biopsy. Loop electroexcision also has excellent success

THE FUTURE: CHEMOPREVENTION

A number of clinical trials are currently underway worldwide to find chemical substances that can stop dysplasia from developing into cancer. Some candidates include antioxidants like vitamin E, vitamin C, and vitamin A, and chemicals called retinoids. Nonsteroidal anti-inflammatory drugs (NSAIDs) such as ibuprofen are also being studied.

A new oral drug, DFMO (difluoromenthylornithine) is currently being studied in clinical trials and shows promise in stopping precancerous cervical cells from developing into cancer. According to University of Texas Anderson Cancer Center researchers, DFMO seems to work by inhibiting the action of a key enzyme that promotes development of cancerous cells.

rates, up to 90 percent; it presents a small risk of narrowing the cervical canal.

Partial hysterectomy is the removal of the uterus, including the cervix; when the fallopian tubes and ovaries are also removed, the procedure is called a complete hysterectomy. The procedure is generally reserved for severely invasive cancer, not dysplasia, but in one study published in 1995, cone biopsies were performed on 1,066 women to remove dysplasia. Of these, 311 underwent hysterectomy within a year. Examination of the removed uterine tissue revealed that only 106 actually had any further dysplasia or cancer.

Natural Healing

Methods that remove dysplasia do not prevent it from recurring. These procedures do not address the most important issue—your general health and the health of the tissues of your cervix, uterus, and vagina. Making a firm commitment to long-term health is an essential investment in a healthy future.

Of all the things you can do to reduce your risk of cervical dysplasia, and your risk of the condition progressing if you have it already, quitting smoking is the most important. If you quit smoking, your risk for rapidly developing dysplasia or cancer can drop by half in mere weeks. In one study, the size of cervical lesions was reduced by at least 20 percent in most of the women who had not smoked for at least six months.

Daily walking or another form of exercise that stimulates deep breathing greatly increases the circulation of life-giving oxygen and blood. Stimulating cardiovascular exercise also increases the strength of the immune system. Aerobic exercise such as dance is a great way to boost circulation and stay in shape at the same time. How about taking a belly-dancing class? This dance form stretches and tones pelvic muscles. Also helpful are stretches such as yoga and gentler exercises designed to move energy through your entire body, such as tai chi.

Dietary Changes

Much research has been done on cervical dysplasia and the levels of nutrients present in the women who have it, and many physicians are recommending these supplements to their patients. Lower-than-normal levels of several nutrients—vitamin C, folic acid, and selenium—are commonly found in women with cervical dysplasia. Recent research indicates that insufficient dietary vitamin A, vitamin C, folic acid, riboflavin, and vitamin E are also strongly associated with the condition.

Folic acid supplementation of 10 mg daily has been associated with improved Pap smears in dysplasia patients.

A lack of vitamin A has long been known to correlate with cervical dysplasia. More recently, high blood levels of vitamin A or retinol, which is formed from carotenoids by the liver, have been associated with cases of dysplasia that go into regression. Lycopene, another carotenoid found in both fresh and cooked tomatoes, also seems to have a protective effect against dysplasia. Topical retinoic acid has also been used to treat the condition.

Whenever you are trying to strengthen your immune system, avoid fried food, caffeine-containing foods and beverages, and refined sugar in any form. These can increase internal heat, or inflammation, and reduce immune function. Inflammation is closely associated with free radicals, which are also thought to be involved in the creation of abnormal cells that may develop into tumors.

Another way to assist your body's cleansing is to normalize the microflora in your intestines by eating fermented foods such as yogurt and sauerkraut. Taking acidophilus supplements to encourage a healthy balance of microflora helps, too.

In addition to adding the above nutrients to the diet, you may wish to try treating the cervix directly with herbs. Naturopathic doctors can

SUPPLEMENTS FOR CERVICAL DYSPLASIA

If you have cervical dysplasia or risk factors associated with it, we recommend the following dietary guidelines.

Folic acid 400 to 600 mcgs to 10 mg daily. Sources: green leafy vegetables, soy products, and whole grains

Riboflavin 1.6 to 10 mg daily. Sources: almonds, wheat germ, and whole grains

Vitamin A, beta-carotene 5,000 to 10,000 IU daily. Sources: red peppers, yams, and green leafy vegetables. Caution: Take no more than 10,000 IU of vitamin A per day; above that level, it could be toxic. Beta-carotene, a water-soluble precursor of vitamin A, is safer

Lycopene 1 to 5 mg daily. Sources: tomatoes and tomato products

Vitamin C 1 to 2 g daily. Sources: fresh fruit

Vitamin E 400 to 800 IU daily. Sources: whole grains, wheat germ oil, seeds

Zinc 15 to 25 mg daily. Sources: whole grains, apples, black-eyed peas

"paint" the cervix with an herbal solution that causes the cervical lining to slough away, much as occurs following cryotherapy. More visits to the doctor are required, however. A home alternative is to use suppositories, although you probably will have to make your own (a recipe is included below), or you can soak a tampon in a strong herbal tea before using.

Herbal Healing

Several categories of herbs are important for treating cervical dysplasia. Although the role that hormones play in promoting dysplasia is not well established by science, we feel that the intricate interplay of these chemicals is an important part of any woman's condition. Therefore, herbs such as the hormone balancer vitex are crucial to any regimen of herbs for healing dysplasia. Liver-supporting herbs help keep excess estrogen from causing damage. And herbs that boost the immune system are obviously necessary.

These categories of herbs—hormone balancers, immune boosters, and others—are known as action types; the herbs we recommend for cervical dysplasia are listed by these categories. We've also included several recipes that combine herbs from each group. You may also design your own herbal formula—simply select one herb from each action type. Each herb has a number of different effects; some may be easier for you to obtain than others, or available in better quality—perhaps some are even growing in your own home garden. Or you may simply feel an attraction to a particular herb. Go ahead and trust your intuition or experience in herbal fields such as Traditional Chinese Medicine or Ayurveda.

Obtain each herb in dried form if you wish to make a tea, or tinctures if you wish to take your herbs in liquid form. You'll want to blend two parts of the hormone-balancing herb and one part of the herbs from the other categories. Tablets and capsules can be taken, too.

If you're making a tea, you may need to separate your herbs into those that are roots, berries, or barks, and those that are leaves, flowers, or other above-ground plant parts. The roots, berries, and barks can be simmered to make a decoction, or strong tea. Bring about six cups of water to a boil and add a 1/4 to a 1/2 cup of herbs; simmer for about twenty minutes, let cool and strain. For leaves and flowers, make an infusion by pouring boiling water over the herbs and letting them steep for about five minutes in a covered teapot or mug. You can also find tablets and tinctures of the herbs mentioned here.

Several of the herbs in these categories can be incorporated into your normal cooking routine. Turmeric and ginger, for example, add flavor to almost any soup, stew, or rice dish. Shiitake mushrooms are available in many grocery stores and are easy to add. Milk-thistle seeds can be powdered in a mortar and pestle, food processor, or coffee grinder and sprinkled on hot or cold cereal or pilafs. Burdock root can be cooked as you would a turnip or parsnip, or mixed with other cooked vegetables. Dandelion greens can be added to salads or steamed with other greens. You can simply eat artichokes. Opt for the organically grown kind if you can.

A Word About Dosage

Unless otherwise indicated, take one-quarter to one-third ounce of the following herbs, per day, in decoction or infusion. If you are using a prepared formula, follow the directions on the package.

Hormone Regulators

Herbs that can increase progesterone, regulate estrogen levels, and reduce prolactin levels may be especially useful for helping to prevent dysplasia and cancer; they have a balancing effect on hormones.

Vitex berries. Usually considered the herb of choice for treating cervical dysplasia.

Black cohosh. This hormone balancer offers mild sedative and anti-inflammatory properties.

Healthy Liver Herbs

Many cancers are a response to a continual irritant that stimulates the abnormal growth of cells. Such irritants include cigarette smoke, the body's own waste products, waste products of disease-causing bacteria and other organisms, and environmental toxins such as pesticides. The inability of the body to break down and get rid of toxic waste products with liver-produced enzymes has been linked to an increased chance of developing cervical dysplasia and cancer. Equally important is the liver's ability to break down and regulate hormones such as estrogen.

Several herbs and foods help the liver and other organs in detoxifying the body. To cleanse the liver, try:

Burdock root. One of the foremost detoxifying herbs.

Dandelion root. This well-known and safe diuretic helps maintain potassium levels while eliminating excess fluid from the body.

Yellow dock root. Another popular cleansing herb, this root also helps boost iron absorption.

Boldo leaves. This South American herb stimulates bile flow.

Artichoke leaf. This popular Mediterranean plant has bile-promoting qualities.

For liver support, try the following herbal remedies:

Milk-thistle seeds. Take two to three capsules or tablets per day of a standardized extract.

Turmeric. This spice, common in Indian and some Mediterranean food, is not only good for you, it's tasty. Take two to four capsules or tablets per day of a standardized extract, or add 1/4 ounce of the rhizome powder or pieces to tea, soups, or stews.

Ginger. This warming herb helps remove stagnation, strengthen digestion and settle the stomach. Take several slices of the fresh root per day in a strong decoction or in other cooked foods—or take four to five capsules daily of the powdered root.

Blood Detoxifiers and Immune Stimulants

These herbs encourage the removal of toxic waste products in the blood.

Red clover flowers. This common American forage plant is a traditional blood tonic.

Echinacea leaves or root. This native American plant is a superior immune booster.

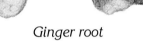

Ginger root

Sarsaparilla root. This original flavoring for root beer is cleansing and detoxifying.

Chaparral leaf. Take 1 tablespoon a day of the finely chopped herb in an infusion or light decoction. Caution: Use for up to two weeks only, and not at all if you have hepatitis or cirrhosis.

Immune Tonics

The following herbs help support the immune system in its effort to recognize abnormal cells and eliminate them from the body. If you wish to use them in liquid extract form, take three to four droppersful three times per day. If you are taking these herbs in capsules or tablets, take two pills, three times daily.

Astragalus. Use prepared root slices in decoction.

Ligustrum berries. This herb blends well with astragalus.

Reishi mushrooms. Make the dried, fruiting body into a decoction.

Fresh or dried shiitake mushrooms. Take 1/3 ounce in decoction—or add three to four fresh mushrooms per day to soups and stews. These are also available in tablet or extract form.

Immune Toning Tea

This tea combines vitex with sarsaparilla to detoxify the blood, astragalus to support the immune system, dandelion to cleanse the liver, and ginger to support it. The vitex makes this tea a complete formula but also affects its otherwise good flavor. You may wish to make the tea without vitex and take vitex in tincture or capsule form instead.

1 teaspoon sarsaparilla root
1 teaspoon astragalus root
1 teaspoon dandelion root
1 teaspoon ginger root
2 teaspoons vitex berries, optional
2 cups water

Heat the herbs in the water at a very low simmer for 5 to 10 minutes. Turn off the heat and let the mixture steep for about 15 minutes. Strain and drink, or store in the refrigerator for up to 3 days.

Cervical Dysplasia Tea

This tea combines vitex to regulate estrogen and progesterone, burdock and milk thistle to cleanse and protect the liver, red clover to cleanse the blood, and astragalus to boost the immune system. Add stevia for sweetness and or mint for flavor, if you wish. You can also blend prepared tinctures of these herbs in the same proportions.

2 teaspoons vitex berries
1 teaspoon burdock root
1 teaspoon red clover
1 teaspoon astragalus root
1/2 teaspoon or more stevia for sweetness, if desired
1/2 to 1 teaspoon peppermint, spearmint, or wintergreen, if desired
5 cups water

Bring herbs and water to a boil. Simmer gently for 5 minutes. Cover pot and let steep 20 more minutes. Strain out herbs. Store in refrigerator up to 3 days; drink 2 to 3 cups per day before meals.

Phytoestrogens

These are herbs that have a mild estrogenic effect in the body. They prevent your own estrogen from overstimulating sensitive tissue, reducing the risk of developing cancer.

Red clover. If you don't wish to use tea, there are commercial preparations that contain this herb.

Kudzu root. Use this Chinese herb in tea or tincture form.

Aromatherapy and Hydrotherapy

Sitz baths with essential oils can help boost circulation and eliminate waste products and toxins from the body's cells. A sitz bath is a bath in which you switch from hot water to cold and back again. To do one, you'll need your bathtub and a second tub, large enough to sit in, for cold water. First move the cold tub into the bathroom and fill it with cold water. Then run water as hot as is comfortable into the bathtub, until it is at least deep enough to reach your navel while you are seated. For an additional circulation boost, add six drops of essential oil of rosemary, cypress, or juniper. Aromatherapists often use geranium and rose to relieve uterine and associated problems. They have the added benefit of relaxing the mind and are thought to promote hormonal and emotional balance. Soak in the warm water for five to ten minutes; then switch to the cold tub for at least a minute. Repeat two to five times. Take a sitz bath up to several times per week. The following recipes using essential oils may also help.

Tampon Soak

If you can, choose pure cotton tampons sold in natural products stores. Be sure to purchase tampons that come enclosed in a cylinder cartridge; the other types will expand and soften too much.

1 heaping teaspoon dried calendula flowers
1 heaping tablespoon dried plantain leaf
1/2 teaspoon Oregon grape root powder
5 drops tea tree essential oil
1 cup distilled water

Put herbs in large pot with water and bring to a boil. Turn off heat and let steep, covered, about 30 minutes. Strain out herb and discard. Add tea tree oil and mix well. Soak tampon in liquid, stirring well to distribute the oil. Use the tampon in the usual way.

Cervical Dysplasia Suppositories

Making suppositories is easy, although finding a mold may call for some ingenuity. Small ice-cube trays work well.

1 tablespoon calendula flowers (15 ml)
1 teaspoon Oregon grape root (5 ml)
1 teaspoon bayberry bark (5 ml)
6 drops tea tree essential oil
1 ounce cocoa butter (30 ml)

Grind the herbs in a coffee grinder or blender. Over low heat, melt cocoa butter in a double boiler until it liquifies. Stir in herbs. Keep on very low heat for at least three hours.

Strain out the herbs and discard. Pour the oil into molds. Cool. When the suppositories are solid, pop them out of the mold and store in a bag in the freezer up to one year.

Insert one suppository deep into the vagina each morning and each evening. It is best to lie down for at least a half hour after inserting the suppository to retain its healing benefits.

CHAPTER 13

SPECIAL SECTION ON PREGNANCY

Many books cover natural pregnancy and birth in greater detail than is possible here. We've asked Raven Lang, a midwife and licensed acupuncturist, the founder of a midwifery school and several associations and the author of three books on natural birth, to give a brief overview of the benefits of natural care for common complaints of pregnancy and birth.

Having a baby is hard work—and at the same time, it is natural work. All over the world, 90% of births take place safely, without medical intervention. But women do need all the help, support, and education they can get for the process of bringing new life into the world. Pregnancy is a time of receptivity, of embracing. Gather your support group of spouse, friends, family, health-care practitioners, and let yourself receive what they can offer you. Perhaps the best advice for a pregnant woman is to not worry about being everything to all people while you are making a human being. This task is devotion and love of the dearest order.

What Midwifery Can Offer

Traditionally, women have lived in situations where the knowledge of mothering has been passed from woman to woman, mother to daughter, sister to sister. The modern, medical approach to pregnancy has had much to offer in assisting high-risk or problem pregnancies, but it can also tend to overtreat common problems or discomforts. And it can be a cold and clinical experience. Three decades ago, a revolution in the handling of pregnancy and birthing took place as the legal profession of midwifery was revived. Most midwifery holds to the belief that pregnancy and birth are natural and healthy processes, and that the least invasive methods of care are usually the best. Many midwives are prepared to work in harmony with

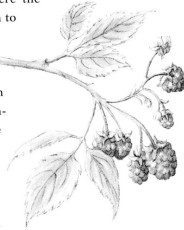

Red Raspberry

your physician and chosen hospital; some are retained as employees by health-care centers.

Midwifery care begins as early in pregnancy as a woman desires, includes labor and delivery, and usually ends somewhere into the child's second month of life. It includes assistance with a wide range of concerns: the mother's health, the baby's health, their psychological and spiritual wellness, and—perhaps most welcome and most ignored by modern medicine—the simple, practical aspects of keeping a home and family together while introducing a new life. Midwifery care does not mean you must have your baby at home; it is often available to women who choose to have their babies in the hospital.

You can find a practicing midwife by simply looking in the yellow pages under midwifery; you can also call your local women's health center, or the Midwives Alliance of North America (see the Resource Directory at the end of this book.) Some states license midwives; some don't. A midwife's training and experience can vary widely, so take your time calling prospective midwives to find one with whom you feel comfortable and secure.

What Traditional Chinese Medicine Can Offer

Traditional Chinese Medicine, including both herbal treatments and acupuncture, can be of immense value to pregnant women. Each pregnancy and each mother is unique; the Chinese system's emphasis on individually tailored treatments can be very effective. Because it is advisable for women to avoid many over-the-counter drugs and antibiotics during pregnancy, alternative treatments can provide great benefits.

Acupuncturists and herbalists who treat pregnant women commonly deal with such problems as anemia, morning sickness, threatened miscarriage, infections, varicose veins, high blood pressure, and pain. Traditional Chinese Medicine can be used to help a potential breech baby turn around for head-first birth. In my practice, I have also seen it effectively induce labor.

This system of medicine is extraordinarily useful in the postpartum period. It can help replenish the energy lost during labor and delivery and restore the mother's strength. It can also help her sleep, establish a full milk supply, or dry up milk if she chooses not to breast-feed.

If you choose to consult a practitioner of Traditional Chinese Medicine, ask about his or her experience treating women during pregnancy and childbirth. Often, your local midwives' association may be able to recommend one.

PREGNANCY, HERBS, AND SAFETY

Perhaps the most important information about herbs and pregnancy is what *not* to take. Many herbs are contraindicated during pregnancy or should be used only under the direction of your health practitioner.

The following herbs are well-known for their safety during pregnancy.

black haw	echinacea	red raspberry leaf
German chamomile	ginger	partridge berry
cramp bark	peppermint	vitex

The following herbs are contraindicated during pregnancy unless recommended by a qualified health-care practitioner. They are safe when used as kitchen spices or in cosmetics.

aloe vera powder	castor	motherwort
angelica	catnip	mugwort
anise	celandine	myrrh
arnica	celery	nutmeg
asafetida	coltsfoot	Oregon grape
ashwaganda	comfrey	osha
barberry	corydalis	parsley
basil	dong quai	pennyroyal
beebalm	elecampane	pleurisy root
black cohosh	ephedra	prickly ash
bladderwrack	fenugreek	quassia
blessed thistle	feverfew	red clover
bloodroot	goldenseal	rue
blue cohosh	guggul	senna
blue flag	horehound	thuja
borage	hyssop	vervain
buchu	ipecac	vitex
bugleweed	juniper	wild indigo
California poppy	lemongrass	wormwood
camphor	licorice	yarrow
cascara sagrada	lobelia	
cassia	mace	

Herbal Healing

There are many herbal remedies that are not only perfectly safe for you and your baby, but wonderfully effective. Here are a few.

Red raspberry. A tea made from this plant's leaves provides extra calcium needed by both mother and fetus. It can also soothe the nervous system, promote sleep, reduce stress, and help muscles recover from hard work—such as labor. It's also inexpensive, readily available, and easily prepared.

Ginger. This common spice is excellent for nausea or morning sickness. Fresh ginger can be sliced and boiled, and the water sipped as a tea throughout the day. If even this tea is unappetizing, try taking powdered ginger as a capsule. For mild symptoms, two capsules of ginger three times a day is adequate. For more severe symptoms, you can go as high as twenty capsules in 24 hours.

Two Chinese formulas commonly used to treat morning sickness are *Pill Curing* and *An Tai Wan.* Morning sickness can be tricky; what might work for one week may cease to work the following week.

CAUTION: For pregnant women whose morning sickness becomes severe and prolonged, it may be necessary to seek the help of a health practitioner. If you are vomiting after every meal for more than a few days, you should contact your health-care professional immediately.

Black haw is excellent for helping the uterus relax, easing premature contractions, and stopping bleeding or spotting. Women with mild symptoms can take two to three capsules three times a day; for stronger symptoms, take three to four capsules four or five times a day. The herb can be taken long-term during pregnancy. Black haw is inexpensive, but you may have to make your own capsules. If you buy it in a powder form, it should be dark and have a strong scent.

Black haw may also be used for painful contractions immediately after delivery, a problem rarely encountered in first-time mothers but frequently during subsequent births. Treatment can be started within minutes after delivery with four capsules, then repeated every several hours for the first day of motherhood.

Valerian is a superior postpartum sleep aid. Because it has a very strong smell and aftertaste, it's best to blend it with other safe, calming herbs, take it with a meal or flavored drink, or take it in capsule form. If you use a tincture made from fresh valerian, you can take 1/2 to 3/4 teaspoon every four hours.

One of the best herbal treatments for postpartum mothers is a hot ginger compress placed on the lower back, breasts, or directly on the perineum. It soothes these sore tissues and helps them relax so that they can heal and strengthen; the aroma of the ginger is soothing to the stomach. To prepare it, you will need a good supply of clean cloth or toweling (large but thin bath-size towels are best for a breast poultice). A crock pot or slow cooker is also helpful; that way, you can keep the herbal broth hot and use the poultice as needed.

Postpartum Compress

3 tablespoons fresh ginger root, chopped fine
2 tablespoons comfrey root, chopped fine
2 tablespoons comfrey leaf or fresh plantain leaf, chopped
8 cups or more water

Simmer roots in a large pot for at least a half hour. Add the comfrey leaves or plantain leaves and turn the heat to low. Steep for at least 10 minutes.

Immerse a clean diaper or towel into the hot mix, wring, and apply to the vulva and perineum. (You may be surprised at how much heat this part of your body can take; you may want to protect your hands with dishwashing gloves when dunking and wringing the towel.) When the cloth cools, repeat the process for up to 20 minutes. Use several times a day during the first postpartum week.

If treating an engorged breast, use a thin bath towel. Wrap the towel completely around the breasts and under the armpit. Repeat until the breast is pink with heat; use as needed. This poultice soothes sore breasts and may help prevent mastitis.

The brew can be reheated and reused, or kept simmering in a crock pot for up to two days—but be sure to use a clean cloth with each application.

Pregnant Belly Oil

To prevent help prevent stretch marks, massage this tried-and-true oil into your belly at least once a day during pregnancy.

4 400-IU vitamin E capsules
4 ounces almond oil or light vegetable oil
1/2 ounce cocoa butter
5 drops lavender essential oil (optional)

Open the vitamin E capsules with a pin and squeeze into the almond oil. Melt the mixture in a saucepan over low heat. Add the cocoa butter. Once the mixture has melted, remove from heat and allow to cool. Add the essential oil and stir; store away from light and heat. Pregnant women can be very sensitive to scents; if you are one of them, simply omit the lavender oil.

betes, gross obesity, and gallbladder or liver disease. Hormone replacement therapy may help prevent heart disease, probably by helping to increase HDL, the so-called "good" cholesterol, and by lowering total cholesterol and LDL, the "bad" cholesterol. Some research suggests that it may also have a direct antioxidant effect on the walls of blood vessels.

Many physicians, aware of the risks of estrogen replacement therapy, are trying much lower doses of estrogen that seem to have few negative side effects. Research is ongoing on the long-term results of such therapy. Prescribing it is a complicated matter of taking many variables into account, such as the type and dose of estrogen prescribed, whether progestins or progesterone are added and how much, the woman's family health history, and her own health factors. Hormone replacement therapy may relieve many menopausal symptoms, such as hot flashes and vaginal dryness. On the other hand, we believe that it should not be prescribed when these symptoms are minor or moderate, because they can be easily addressed by natural healing methods—with much less risk.

Side Effects

Women taking estrogen supplements worry most about increased risk of endometrial or breast cancer. Most of the time, estrogen is prescribed with progesterone, which reduces the risk of endometrial cancer sharply, but probably not breast cancer. Studies of breast cancer and estrogen therapy remain inconclusive, but a Swedish study found a

ESTROGEN REPLACEMENT: RISKS AND BENEFITS

Benefits

Reduced severity and number of hot flashes

Reduced risk of cardiovascular disease

Reduced severity of osteoporosis; reduced risk of osteoporosis-related fractures

Slows thinning, weakening, and drying of vaginal walls

Slows weakening of urinary tissues, preventing some kinds of incontinence

Decreases depression

Risks

(Many of the following symptoms do not occur with low-dose estrogen replacement therapy.)

Breast cancer

Breast enlargement and tenderness

Fibrocystic breast disease

Cyclic bleeding; breakthrough bleeding

Gallstones

Nausea or vomiting

Cramps, bloating, or other menstrual discomfort

High blood pressure and increased clotting

Acne

Altered libido

moderately increased risk of breast cancer after more than ten years of estrogen supplementation. Those who also took progestin had even higher risk.

NATURAL HEALING

A healthy lifestyle helps the body weather almost any change or challenge. Though overall risk of heart disease and osteoporosis rises after menopause, women at risk can take steps to increase their chances of enjoying a vital, strong old age. And despite a family history of difficult menopause, there are healing strategies specific to menopause that can help many women defy genetics.

A recent study compared vaginal epithelium cells from 1,638 healthy, postmenopausal nonsmokers with those from 531 similar women who smoke. Researchers found that the smokers had a higher rate of cell changes suggesting vaginal atrophy than the nonsmokers; in addition, the smokers reached menopause an average of two years earlier (at a mean age of 48.5 years) than the nonsmokers.

Some research has shown that exercise can eliminate or lessen hot flashes. Women responding to the Kronenberg survey of 2,000 women had fewer menopausal problems when they exercised at least three times a week. A Swedish study of 79 postmenopausal women compared those who chose exercise instead of hormone replacement therapy to a control group of nearly 900 women. The women who spent about three and a half hours per week exercising had no hot flashes whatsoever, including the women who had suffered from them before they began working out. More moderate exercisers had fewer and milder hot flashes. Other studies on exercise and women just entering menopause report that exercise has a similar effect, regardless of whether a woman is taking supplemental estrogen.

Sex, in addition to being good exercise, may beneficially influence hormonal levels. One study finds that women who have frequent sex tend to have fewer hot flashes, although this may simply mean that women who have hot flashes naturally have less desire to have sex. Noted sex researchers William Masters and Virginia Johnson found that some women who engaged in regular sex preserved their vaginal muscle tone and lubrication into their 70s.

As for urinary continence, one particular exercise, the Kegel exercise, can be helpful. To perform the Kegel exercise, simply use the same muscle action you would to stop urinating in midstream. Repeat the contractions, first slowly and then rapidly, up to 100 times. Then hold the contractions for 10 seconds This exercise can be done anywhere, anytime; it's the same one postpartum women use to regain pelvic muscle tone.

Dietary Strategies

According to the Kronenberg survey of 2,000 women, those women whose diet is low in fat have even fewer symptoms of menopause than those who exercise regularly, although women who eat well may have a healthier lifestyle in general. Be that as it may, a low-fat, high-fiber diet certainly can't hurt.

Foods to include in that diet include linolenic acid, the essential fatty acid found in flaxseed oil and evening primrose oil, and the omega-3 fatty acids found in salmon, trout, and mackerel. These oils help keep skin, hair, and vaginal tissues healthy. Flaxseed also contains lignans, which have both anticancer and estrogen-like properties.

Phytoestrogens and Menopause

A growing body of evidence suggests that phytoestrogens—plant compounds that mimic estrogen in the body—can benefit women before, during, and after menopause. Two particular substances, the isoflavones genistein and daidzein, act as weak estrogens, occupying the molecular niches that estrogen normally settles in, and stimulating those tissues more gently and evenly than the body's own estrogen. In women who are years away from menopause, these compounds may ease the effects of excess estrogen that are responsible for PMS, endometriosis, uterine fibroids, and other abnormal tissue growth, In menopausal women, phytoestrogens can buffer the symptoms of a dwindling estrogen supply.

Soybeans and some soy products are probably the best-known sources of phytoestrogens. But James A. Duke, Ph.D., an internationally respected herbalist, recommends a host of other phytoestrogen sources. Yellow lentils, black (turtle) beans, lima beans, anasazi beans, red kidney beans, and red lentils actually contain more genistein than soybeans. Black-eyed peas,

SOY AND HEALTH STATISTICS

Daily Phytoestrogen Intake

North American women	5 grams
Asian	30–100 mg
Japanese	200 mg

Percentage of Menopausal Women Reporting Hot Flashes

European	70–80 percent
American	58 percent
Chinese	18 percent
Singaporean	14 percent

Sources: Boulet et al, 1994; Cassidy et al, 1993; Coward et al, 1993; Greendale & Judd, 1995; Tang, 1994; Wilcox et al, 1995

mung, and adzuki beans have almost as much genistein as soybeans, while fava and great northern beans have about 80 percent as much. In fact, all legumes are high in isoflavones.

Dietary Supplements

Back in 1937, Dr. Evan Shute, a pioneer in vitamin E therapy, wrote about how well it relieved menopausal symptoms. A few years later, the prominent British researcher Dr. Hugh McLaren said that vitamin E improves the strength and flexibility of the vagina and heals abrasions. He predicted that someday doctors would turn to vitamin E because estrogen would be found to be carcinogenic.

Several clinical studies in the late 1940s confirmed vitamin E's abilities. Dr. Rita Finkler's study of sixty-six menopausal women found that thirty-one experienced "good to excellent relief" from symptoms. For another sixteen women, improvement was fair. This was with relatively low doses of 20 to 100 IU daily. When the vitamin was replaced with a placebo, symptoms in seventeen of the women quickly returned. Vitamin E causes very few negative side effects, and benefits both the cardiovascular system and the brain. New studies of the use of vitamin E for menopausal symptoms are currently under way, and dozens of women back them with their personal success stories.

Women should also consider supplements to prevent osteoporosis. Calcium, magnesium, and vitamin D are important, and silica and boron may be added as well.

Herbal Healing

The most popular herbs used to ease symptoms of menopause are black cohosh, vitex, dong quai, and ginseng. Evidence is mounting that these herbs also exert a myriad of protective effects on the body. They belong to several categories of herbs that are helpful in menopause: hormone regulators; adrenal support herbs for the glands that produce hormones; relaxing herbs; mood lifters; tonics for the blood, uterine tissues, and urinary tract; and cooling herbs to help fend off hot flashes.

You can design your own herbal program for menopause by choosing an herb or two from each of the following categories, based on your needs.

Herbs that contain phytoestrogens. These herbs help balance hormones—they stimulate production when hormone levels are low, and moderate them when they are high. The most effective herbs for hormone regulation are black cohosh and vitex, an ancient Mediterranean herb that increases natural progesterone levels. Clinical studies demonstrate that both herbs relieve menopausal symptoms. Also recommended are red clover, red Korean or red Chinese ginseng. Since 1956, about 1.5 million menopausal women in Germany have used black cohosh, which is prescribed by European doctors and sold in drug stores there. The herb relieves some menopausal symptoms without raising risks of breast cancer and is effective against stress-related menopausal problems.

Adrenal support herbs. These herbs help support the adrenals in their job of building estrogen. Traditional Chinese Medicine calls them kidney tonics. They include eleuthero, also known as Siberian ginseng; American ginseng; and the Chinese herbs rehmannia, psoralea, and ligustrum. Also included in this category are reishi mushrooms. These helpful substances can help relieve night sweats and fatigue.

Relaxing herbs. This category includes California poppy, valerian, hops, kava kava, passion flower, and linden flower. These herbs can help create a feeling of ease and promote refreshing sleep.

Mood lifters. St. John's wort (discussed in detail in Mood Disorders) and ginkgo, which also boosts circulation to the brain, are the best mood lifters to use for menopause.

GLORIOUS GINSENG

The Chinese often recommend ginseng for women over forty. Robert Atkins, M.D., author of *Dr. Atkins' New Diet Revolution*, noticed that about four-fifths of his patients complaining of hot flashes responded to red Chinese ginseng (*Panax ginseng*) in two to six weeks. Ginseng may help increase libido and energy, alleviate depression, and stabilize blood pressure and sugar levels. Some Chinese studies suggest that it encourages cell growth and may help protect against cancer. It is a strong antioxidant, and contains small amounts of important nutrients, such as vitamins A, B2, B6, B12, calcium, iron, folic acid, magnesium, zinc, and pantothenic acid.

Blood tonics. Yellow dock root, nettle leaf, and dong quai can help the body build strong blood, which helps nourish the skin and other tissues that tend to become dryer during menopause. Dong quai's reputation in Asia as a beneficial herb is probably second only to that of ginseng. Be aware that dong quai can increase bleeding, so if long and heavy periods are part of your menopausal symptoms, choose other blood tonics such as nettles or yellow dock.

Uterine tonics. Dong quai, red raspberry leaf, and motherwort help maintain healthy tissues, especially uterine tissues. See the caution about dong quai under blood tonics.

Urinary tract tonics. Herbs in this category help support healthy bladder and urinary tract tissues. They include saw palmetto, goldenrod, marshmallow root, and nettle leaf

Cooling herbs. Licorice, elder and linden flowers, honeysuckle, yarrow, and hibiscus can help to reduce hot flashes.

There are many ways to combine these herbs into formulas. Dr. Lois Johnson, who for seven years has used herbs to treat her patients' menopausal complaints, recommends an herb tea of schisandra berries, hibiscus, linden, lemon balm, and sage to cool down hot flashes. If night sweats or insomnia are factors, she adds skullcap or motherwort.

Brian Weissbuch, a licensed acupuncturist with twenty-eight years experience, says that at least 80 percent of his menopausal patients find that herbs can relieve their symptoms. About half find that some symptoms, such as vaginal dryness, improve immediately. He recommends starting on herbal therapy when menopause symptoms first appear. Weissbuch customizes his formulas to the individual, but usually starts with black cohosh and red raspberry leaf.

He also emphasizes that if you are currently on hormone replacement therapy and wish to replace it with an herbal formula, it is crucial to make a gradual transition. "Take small doses of herbs at first, gradually increasing the dose, and then begin phasing out the hormones in the second month," he says.

Dr. Lois Johnson's Hot-Flash Tea

This tea can be sipped throughout the day to relieve hot flashes. Adding the lemon juice makes it even more cooling.

2 teaspoons schisandra berries
1 teaspoon hibiscus flowers
1/2 teaspoon linden flowers
1/2 teaspoon lemon balm
1/2 teaspoon sage
lemon juice (optional)
1 quart water

Bring water to a boil. Remove from heat; add herbs and steep for 15 minutes. Strain out herbs; store for up to 3 days in the refrigerator. This tea can be drunk cool or hot.

Menopause Tincture

Try this blend of tinctures to relieve hot flashes and vaginal dryness.

1 teaspoon black cohosh tincture
1 teaspoon vitex tincture
1/2 teaspoon ginseng tincture
1/2 teaspoon licorice root tincture
1/2 teaspoon dong quai tincture
1/2 teaspoon motherwort tincture

Blend the tinctures. Take 1/2 teaspoon in a little water three times daily.

Variations

• To relieve water retention: Add 1 teaspoon dandelion tincture.

• To help protect the heart and blood vessels: add 1 teaspoon tincture of hawthorn berries, leaves, flowers, or a combination.

• To ease depression or anxiety: Add 1 teaspoon St. John's wort tincture or California poppy tincture, or 1/2 teaspoon of each.

This recipe can also be made as a tea; substitute dried herbs in the same proportions. Simmer the herbs in a quart of water for about 10 minutes, then remove from heat and let them steep for another 15. Drink 1 cup morning and evening.

Aromatherapy

Several essential oils can be helpful during menopause. These include clary sage, anise, fennel, cypress, angelica, coriander, sage, peppermint, lemon, and, to a lesser degree, basil. All help relieve hot flashes. Sage is one of the most useful. It has an age-old reputation for lessening excessive sweating and can also check hot flashes and keep them away for hours. You can receive the benefits of these herbs in massage oil or a fragrant bath. Don't use sage essential oil if you have epilepsy or seizures.

Essential oils of geranium, rose, and orange blossom, also known as neroli, are considered hormone balancers. Europeans have long used them in face creams to smooth wrinkles. They also smell divine. Added to vitamin E oil, these essential oils may help heal vaginal abrasions that can occur during intercourse. They also can be added to a ready-made cream, lotion, or salve. If you choose to add essential oils to ready-made products, be sure to purchase products that contain healthy, nonirritating ingredients with no synthetic essential oils. Be aware that any product containing vegetable or petroleum oil can break down the latex in a condom or diaphragm.

Meanwhile, for emotional symptoms of menopause, use the fragrances of chamomile, jasmine, and neroli as a perfume, massage oil, or room freshener, or place a dab of one or all on a small cloth or handkerchief and carry it with you. These fragrances are well-known mood enhancers.

Menopause Massage and Body Oil

6 drops lemon oil
5 drops geranium oil
2 drops clary sage oil
1 drop angelica oil
1 drop jasmine oil
2 ounces vegetable oil such as almond oil or body lotion

Combine the ingredients. Use at least once a day as a massage oil or lotion, or add two teaspoons to bath water. Adding essential oils to a commercial lotion makes a less oily formula.

Rejuvenation Oil

2 ounces almond oil (or any vegetable oil)
6 drops rose geranium essential oil
6 drops lavender essential oil
1 drop neroli essential oil (optional)
Vitamin E oil capsules to total about 1500 IU, opened

Combine ingredients. Apply to the labia or vagina as needed.

CHAPTER 15

HEART DISEASE

*After age 65, one in three women has some form
of heart disease. The good news is that natural healing
methods can almost always help.*

Imagine this scene: You are sitting at an outdoor cafe. People are passing by; it's a beautiful day. Suddenly, the person at the table next to you gasps and falls to the ground, fists to chest. Somebody shouts, "Call a doctor, heart attack!"

Did you see a man or a woman as the victim? Most people picture a man having a heart attack.

When the American Heart Association commissioned a survey of 1,000 women older than 25, only 8 percent considered heart disease and stroke their most serious health threat. The majority of those surveyed were right—unless the woman is age 65 or older, when one in three women has heart disease. The overall leading cause of death in women, heart disease kills 250,000 American women per year.

Some doctors and researchers believe that estrogen may be responsible for protecting women from heart disease until menopause. However, more post-menopausal women are seeking alternatives to hormone replacement therapy because of its side effects—an increase in the risk of breast and endometrial cancers, among others. Researchers have found that adding progesterone to estrogen eliminates the increased risk of endometrial cancer, but have not yet resolved the riddle of breast-cancer risk. For some women with a family history of the disease, the reduced risk of osteoporosis and heart disease that estrogen offers may not be worth it.

During the last forty years, most clinical and scientific research on heart disease has focused on men. As a result, we know much more about men and heart disease than we do about women and heart disease.

Hawthorn

But we do know that compared to men, women who develop coronary artery disease are more likely to die from it or suffer a drastic reduction in quality of life. The reason may be that women tend to be older and sicker when they develop heart disease than men. In addition, women often are not treated for heart disease as aggressively as men. The medical treatment of women complaining about chest pain is sometimes delayed and less intensive than men's treatment, even after the women's initial tests indicate problems.

Fortunately, women and their doctors are becoming more aware of the need for including the cardiovascular system in routine health care. Intensive studies of cardiovascular disease in women are ongoing, and the findings will increase our knowledge substantially.

Defining Heart Disease

The heart is a muscle that pumps 100,000 times daily, pushing 2,000 gallons of blood through a range of vessels to deliver nutrients, hormones, and oxygen to every cell in the body. An electrical stimulus prompts the heart's regular beat; its rhythmical contractions push blood through two pumping chambers, two valves, and the pulmonary artery, which carries the blood into the lungs for oxygenation. Oxygenated blood then returns to the heart, where two more chambers pump it through two more valves and the aorta, then out to the body. Because the heart also needs blood for itself, the right and left coronary arteries at the top of the heart provide this supply.

The term "heart disease" encompasses several kinds of problems with the heart and blood vessels; that's why the term cardiovascular disease is used, too. The conditions that are associated with heart disease often have several names, which can make understanding them a frustrating task.

High blood pressure. This is the most common chronic medical condition, affecting 17 to 25 million women or 10 percent of the United States' population. After menopause, it becomes more common among women than men.

Blood pressure itself is a measurement of the pressure blood exerts on the walls of arteries. It is expressed in two numbers, with the top one indicating pressure during the heartbeat, and the bottom one indicating pressure while the heart is at rest. Blood pressure that is always high can damage artery walls.

Cardiac arrhythmia. This term simply means irregular heartbeat. If your heart seems to stop for a minute, then you feel a "thud" in the chest, that may be an arrhythmia. Also known as heart palpitations, these small

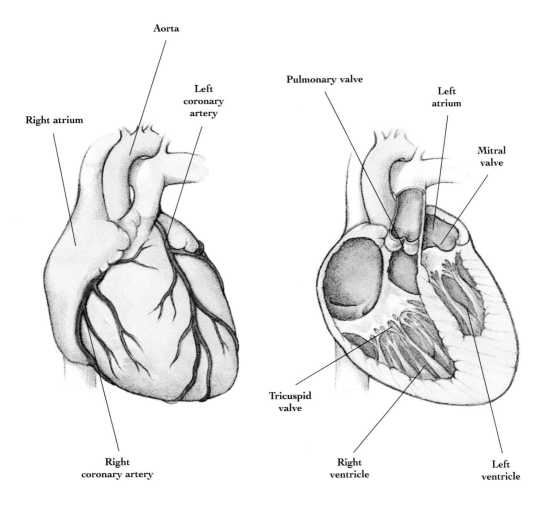

Right atrium

Aorta

Left
coronary
artery

Right
coronary artery

Pulmonary valve

Left
atrium

Mitral
valve

Tricuspid
valve

Right
ventricle

Left
ventricle

Heart anatomy, anterior view

breaks in the heart's rhythm are usually occasional and harmless. Many women feel them during heavy exercise or a hot flash.

Serious arrhythmias may result in dizziness and shortness of breath. Any persistent irregular heartbeat requires consultation with a physician, especially if you have a family history of heart disease.

Heart-valve disease. In the chambers and major blood vessels of the heart are four valves that open as the heart pumps and close as it rests to keep blood flowing in the right direction. Impairment of these valves can result in palpitations, chest pain, easy fatigue, breathlessness, or fainting. Prolapse of the mitral valve, which controls blood flow from the left atrium to the left ventricle, is particularly common in women—about 5 percent have it. The condition is usually benign, but on occasion can be so serious that the valve must be surgically replaced with an artificial one.

Coronary artery disease. Also known as coronary heart disease or coronary atherosclerosis or arteriosclerosis, this is narrowing or hardening of the arteries that crown the heart. It can be present without symptoms until one or both of the arteries is so severely narrowed that an extra burden on the heart—exercise, stress, or other exertion—results in chest pain or sudden heart attack.

Angina. This term refers to chest pains behind the breastbone, sometimes called angina pectoris. When the heart is asked to work harder but can't get enough oxygen to do it, this means that the arteries that carry blood to the heart muscle are narrowed by an accumulation of plaque—the coronary artery disease described above. The attacks usually last for only a few minutes. When chest pain occurs unpredictably and often, it is known as unstable angina—and usually foretells a heart attack.

Heart attack. Also known as myocardial infarction, or literally "heart muscle death," heart attack can be mild, serious, or fatal. Some heart attacks occur without symptoms. When one of the coronary arteries becomes completely blocked by fatty plaque, a blood clot, or a

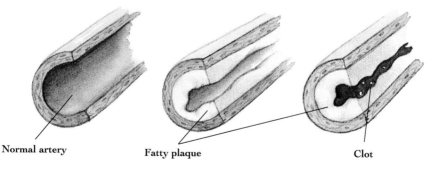

Normal artery   Fatty plaque   Clot

Normal, narrowing and clogged arteries

combination of both, the heart muscle is deprived of oxygen and nutrients; parts of it begin to die. The resulting pain differs from that of angina; it radiates from the chest to the left arm or the neck, jaw, and back. Sweating, nausea, fainting, and a feeling of impending doom may accompany the attack. So-called "silent" heart attacks that occur without symptoms cause damage to the heart, too, but are usually detected only by heart scans or a blood analysis that discovers chemicals released by dying heart tissue.

Congestive heart failure. This condition results from a damaged or weakened heart that can't pump enough blood to keep the body healthy. Congestive heart failure can result from valve disorders, coronary artery disease, chronic high blood pressure, a previous heart attack, or a combination of problems. Symptoms include difficulty breathing, fatigue, and fluid retention, especially in the lungs.

Stroke. Stroke damages the brain, not the heart, but many of its risk factors, preconditions, and mechanisms are the same as those of heart disease. Stroke occurs when a blood vessel in the brain becomes blocked or bursts. The conditions for stroke are the same as those for heart attack: narrowed and/or hardened blood vessels and/or a clot that becomes lodged in the vessel, blocking blood flow to a part of the brain. Stroke can result in paralysis, loss of brain function, or death.

The Cholesterol Connection

Why do arteries become clogged? The stuff that builds up on the inside of arteries, narrowing the channel through which blood flows, is called fatty plaque. It is made of lipids—fats and fat-like substances and fibrous tissue such as collagen. One of the main fat-like substances that builds fatty plaque is cholesterol, that much-talked-about food component often implicated in heart disease.

The artery-clogging buildup can begin at an early age; autopsies of males and females, ages 15 to 34, who were killed in accidents showed that the arteries of many held plaque and fatty deposits. When researchers measured cholesterol levels in the victims' blood, they found that high cholesterol correlated with more lesions, calcium deposits, and artery scarring.

But the role of cholesterol in heart disease is not well-understood, and scientific research into it is ongoing and sometimes contradictory. Cholesterol is found in animal fats and oils but also continuously synthesized by the body. And it apparently plays a very different role in the heart disease of women than it does in men. Research is now focusing on different parts of the cholesterol puzzle. Triglycerides, one of the building blocks of cholesterol, are found in both animal and vegetable fats. High-density lipoprotein, the so-called "good cholesterol" or HDL, contains a higher proportion of proteins to actual cholesterol than low-density lipoprotein, the "bad cholesterol" or LDL. HDL tends to carry cholesterol away from the arteries and back to the liver, where it can be removed from the body. Recent research has focused on pinpointing what kinds of these substances create heart disease under what circumstances. For example, one study in 1988 suggested that even if a woman's total cholesterol level is normal, low HDL levels may indicate her increased risk of coronary artery disease. When the same study compared heart-disease risks in men and women, it found that women younger than 75 usually had a lower risk even at higher total cholesterol levels than men. This implies that for women, a total cholesterol figure may have less meaning than it does for men.

Currently, total cholesterol levels of less than 200 mg/dl are considered to be no cause for alarm, but truly healthy levels may be even lower—146 for total cholesterol and 130 for LDL cholesterol. In our experience, ideal cholesterol levels range from 130 to 160. Unfortunately, a quarter of the adult women in the United States have readings greater than 260 mg/dl.

RISK FACTORS FOR CORONARY ARTERY DISEASE

Family history of the disease

Cigarette smoking

High blood pressure

High total cholesterol, triglycerides, or LDLs; low HDLs

Diabetes

Obesity

High-fat or low-nutrient diet, high sugar intake

Poor responses to stress

Menopause before age 50

Sedentary lifestyle

WHAT A DOCTOR WILL DO

One of the best ways to determine your heart-disease risk is to consider your risk factors, your family's health history, and how sedentary your lifestyle has been. In a regular exam, your doctor should request a complete blood count and examine your cholesterol and triglyceride levels as well as the ratio of HDL to total cholesterol. This ratio may be the measurement that is most predictive of your risk for coronary artery disease. A ratio below 3.5 is thought to be a less-than-average risk; 3.5 to 4.5 is average; and above 4.5 signals higher-than-average risk. The National Cholesterol Education Program recommends that all adults over 20 should have a total cholesterol measurement every 5 years. Many communities and public health clinics offer free or low-cost tests.

If your total cholesterol is borderline to high (200–239 mg/dl) and your HDL cholesterol is greater than 35, you should be checked more frequently. Other tests your doctor may order include blood pressure, exercise electrocardiogram, exercise echocardiography, radioisotope scans, fluoroscopic examinations, magnetic resonance imaging, and angiocardiography.

Physicians also are very much aware that lifestyle affects heart disease; research has long supported the efficacy of increasing exercise, managing stress, quitting smoking, and cutting cholesterol. Doctors almost always recommend these changes to help you avoid or recover from a heart attack and reduce your risk factors for later problems. A variety of medications may also be prescribed.

Cutting Cholesterol

Treatment goals usually include increasing your level of HDL, the "good cholesterol," and increasing your HDL/total cholesterol ratio. Once a program of lifestyle changes has been in place for three to six weeks, your physician will probably want to retest your cholesterol; a third test is often done at three months. If your cholesterol levels are decreasing, doctors will set up a regular recheck schedule. If not, they may refer you to a dietician. If your levels remain elevated after six months, your physician may recommend drug therapy. Here are the some of the most often-prescribed cholesterol medications, along with some of their common side effects.

Nicotinic acid (niacin) is a B vitamin that lowers LDL cholesterol and raises HDL cholesterol, although it is not known exactly how it works. Niacin is inexpensive and produces few side effects. It can cause minor digestive problems, make the skin itchy and dry, and cause the face and upper body to flush, although this often stops after several weeks of use. Women with peptic ulcer disease, liver disease, or gout should not use it.

Bile acid sequestrants (cholestyramines) bind bile acids in the colon to reduce LDL cholesterol levels. They are available in many forms, including a flavored bar. Side effects can include constipation, bloating, nausea, and gas, as well as interference with absorption of other drugs. When used long-term, these medications can result in deficiencies of fat-soluble vitamins.

Hydroxymethylglutaryl coenzyme A reductase inhibitors (lovastatin, pravastatin) are widely prescribed to prevent the liver from manufacturing cholesterol. In some women, lovastatin reduces LDL cholesterol by 24 to 40 percent. Side effects can include muscle pain, fatigue, insomnia, headaches, rashes, and digestive upsets, but they are usually mild and brief.

Regulating Blood Pressure

Because high blood pressure means the heart is working too hard and possibly damaging blood vessels, the condition is not just a symptom or risk factor, but a problem in itself. Currently, millions of women take blood-pressure medication. These drugs sometimes save lives but can be expensive, and their side effects can reduce the quality of life. Some blood-pressure medications actually increase total and LDL cholesterol levels and reduce HDL levels. Others may cause loss of libido.

Some blood-pressure medications work for some individuals and not others; effective dosage often varies. If you take high-blood-pressure medication, it is extremely important to stay in close touch with your physician and report any side effects immediately.

Usually, a beta-blocker and a diuretic will be the first drugs prescribed. Below is more information about the most common high-blood-pressure drugs:

Diuretics such as furosemide reduce total blood volume and lower overall blood pressure by increasing urine output. They can deplete electrolytes such as calcium and magnesium and interfere with sexual function.

Beta-blockers. This large family of drugs includes propranolol, sold under the trade name Inderal. Beta-blockers calm the beta-adrenergic system, a partnership between the nervous and hormonal systems, by decreasing the rate and force of the heart's contractions. In angina

ESTROGEN SUPPLEMENTATION

Estrogen replacement therapy is commonly prescribed to prevent cardiovascular disease. In fact, even women who report no or few menopausal complaints often find their doctors suggesting estrogen to fend off the possibility of future heart problems. Women who take estrogen are estimated to have one-third the incidence of cardiovascular disease of women who do not. The Harvard Nurses' Health Study of 48,000 women reported 50 percent fewer heart attacks in women who took estrogen; such women also tend to have better health, diet, and medical care than others.

How estrogen protects the heart is not completely clear. It is thought to improve a woman's ability to metabolize fats and cholesterol by raising HDL, the "good cholesterol," and decreasing LDL. However, it is one of the most controversial areas of women's health. The Menopause chapter treats this subject in more detail.

patients, beta-blockers reduce the oxygen requirements of the heart muscle, allowing it to function on a reduced blood flow. For patients who have already had a heart attack, beta-blockers can increase survival rates.

These drugs, however, can have dangerous side effects, including nervous system disturbances such as insomnia, fatigue, and lethargy. In rare cases, they can have more severe consequences, such as decreasing HDL cholesterol levels. In patients with congestive heart failure, their use requires close monitoring.

Angiotensin converting enzyme (ACE) inhibitors. These drugs reduce blood pressure by dilating the arteries and reducing fluid volume. They have fewer side effects than beta-blockers: a chronic dry, irritating cough; rashes; edema; and, in some patients with kidney disease, kidney failure.

Calcium channel blockers. These drugs, with trade names including Verapamil, Isoptin, and Calan, also dilate blood vessels. In addition, they decrease the rate and force of the heart muscle's contractions. They can cause headaches, dizziness, and water retention; women with heart failure cannot take them. They are also hard on the liver. A recent report from Sweden suggests that these drugs may increase the risk of depression and suicide more than other antihypertensive medications.

Adrenergic inhibiting agents. This group includes methyldopa, reserpine, and clonidine. These drugs act directly on the brain and spinal cord to reduce blood pressure and are prescribed when other drugs fail. Reserpine is the least expensive because it is a naturally occurring alkaloid from the snake root plant (*Rauwolfia serpentaria*).

Medical Treatments for Other Heart Conditions

Treatment for angina usually starts with a beta-blocker. A nitroglycerin tablet can be placed under the tongue for nearly instant relief of chest pain. Long-acting nitrate drugs are sometimes used, but some patients develop a tolerance to them. Sometimes calcium blockers are added to boost effectiveness.

Aspirin helps prevent heart attacks when taken in small daily doses (60 to 150 mg a day) because it slightly inhibits blood clotting. Aspirin is not harmless; it can cause side effects such as liver toxicity and bleeding in the digestive tract. Avoid it if you have high blood pressure, a liver disease such as hepatitis C, or if you smoke cigarettes.

Women with arrhythmias may be prescribed beta-blockers, calcium channel blockers, or sodium channel blockers. Some of them, such as quinidine, procainamide, and lidocaine, slow the speed of nerve conduction through the heart muscle but may also lower the heart's efficiency.

When arrhythmias become life-threatening, a pacemaker can be surgically implanted. These devices are now lighter and smarter than those of a decade ago; some monitor subtle changes in heartbeat and activate only when arrhythmia occurs.

In cases of coronary artery disease or stroke, thrombolytics or other clot-busting drugs may be used. Tissue plasminogen activator, also known as TPA and sold under the name Activase, is often given shortly after a heart attack because it reduces mortality and shortens recovery in some patients. Recent studies show, however, that women do not respond as well to thrombolytics as men.

Digitalis, a natural compound from the common foxglove, is often used in cases of congestive heart failure. A British physician learned from a female herbalist about the beneficial effects of this plant more than 200 years ago; it remains one of the most important drugs for strengthening the heartbeat. Its side effects can include nausea, nerve pain, and mental confusion. It can be deadly if too much builds up in the body. Older women suffer more side effects from digitalis, possibly because their livers may not efficiently remove it from the blood. Caution: Do not pluck foxglove from your garden and try it at home; doing so has killed a number of people.

Surgical Measures

Three surgical procedures are commonly performed to remedy heart disease.

Valve replacement. When a heart valve is damaged or hardened and unable to function normally, it can be replaced with a valve made of metal, plastic, or pig tissue. The success rate of valve replacement is fairly high, but it requires major thoracic surgery and a long recovery.

Angioplasty. This surgery involves threading a catheter with a balloon at the end into a blocked artery. After the balloon is in place, it is inflated, compressing the plaque and opening the passageway. Angioplasty is often successful, but sometimes the blockage returns. Women do not respond to angioplasty as well as men, perhaps because they tend to be older and sicker when the procedure is done or because there are too few studies of women to accurately assess it.

Bypass surgery. As with angioplasty, women do less well with this procedure than men, so it is recommended less often. Bypass surgery is a treatment of last resort: a vein is taken from a leg and grafted onto the narrowed coronary artery to bypass the clogged area. The heart is stopped during the procedure, and a heart-lung machine keeps the body alive. Some say this surgery is done far too often. It also does not remove the causes of blocked coronary arteries.

NATURAL HEALING

Heart disease is a lifestyle illness—in other words, it can be prevented because many of the risk factors can be controlled. Even when a cardiovascular disease is diagnosed, natural healing strategies such as changes in diet, exercise, and herbal regimens can be highly effective.

Cigarette smoking is a major contributor to heart disease. Those who smoke now may find it encouraging that once you quit, your risk of heart disease is half that of those who continue to smoke—regardless of how long you have smoked.

Exercise, even moderate but regular exercise, as little as thirty minutes every day, aids cardiovascular fitness. According to Dr. Claudia Chae, lead researcher of a Harvard Medical School study, exercising often is more important than how long you do it. Although her study was on men, Chae feels that the American Heart Association guidelines of a thirty-minute-plus workout, three or four times a week, which the study results supported, would also benefit women.

In Chae's study, men who exercised once or twice weekly had a 36-percent lower risk of heart disease than nonexercisers. Men who exercised three to four times weekly reduced their risk by 38 percent; those who exercised five times or more weekly reduced their risk by 46 percent. A different study at the University of Pittsburgh Medical Center shows that black women who walk or run reduce their risks of developing high blood pressure after just one week of exercise.

Stress and your reaction to it also play a significant role in heart disease. Research at Duke University Medical Center in Durham, North Carolina, shows that patients with coronary artery disease and angina who learn to manage and release stress reduce their risk of heart attacks or need for cardiac bypass surgery more than patients who receive only standard cardiovascular care.

Dietary Changes

Women want to know whether eating less fat will help reduce their chance of heart problems when they reach their 60s and 70s. Men benefit from reducing fat intake, but questions remain about the relationship of cholesterol to heart disease in women. The American Heart Association and the National Cholesterol Education Program maintain that women should follow the same dietary guidelines as men until proven otherwise. Other expert groups, including the U.S. Preventive Task Force, maintain that women under 45 don't need cholesterol screening. What much research suggests is that a low-fat, high-fiber, natural diet can help improve anyone's overall health.

The diet that doctors recommend for those at risk for heart disease, and anyone seeking to prevent it, restricts fat to less than 30 percent of total daily calories, and saturated fat to below 10 percent. Cholesterol consumption should be less than 300 mg daily. An even more restrictive diet cuts saturated fat to less than 7 percent of calories per day and cholesterol to under 200 mg per day.

It's possible to eat well on such a diet. The two most proven cuisines for heart health are Mediterranean foods based on grains, vegetables, fish, olive oil, and some red wine; and a very low-fat, Asian-influenced diet based on tofu, sea vegetables such as nori and kelp, aduki and mung beans, and rice. A study done in Lyon, France shows that fatal recurrences of heart attacks drop by half when subjects adopt a Mediterranean diet.

Both the Mediterranean and Asian diets are rich in soluble and insoluble fibers, B vitamins, antioxidant vitamins, flavonoids, and healthy amino acids like arginine. Arginine is a precursor of nitric oxide, which can help normalize blood pressure. Vitamins B6, B12, and folic acid help metabolize and lower sulfur amino acids like methionine and homocysteine, which have been linked with a higher risk of coronary artery disease. Tofu and other bean products contain genistein, phytoestrogens, and other nutrients that have protective effects on the heart.

A mostly vegetarian version of these diets may confer even more benefits. Vegetarians have a much lower rate of heart disease than omnivores, probably because they eat far fewer saturated fats and less cholesterol. In addition, the estrogen-like compounds in soy products help prevent heart attacks and strokes. A recent review of 38 volunteer studies suggests that when soy protein is substituted for animal protein, levels of total cholesterol, LDL cholesterol, and triglycerides decline while HDL levels stay the same. Benefits were seen with as little as 30 grams of soy a day, which is about 2 cups of soy milk or 2/3 cup cubed tofu. The volunteers with the highest pre-study cholesterol readings reaped the greatest benefits.

Foods for a Healthy Heart

Fruits and vegetables lowered subjects' heart-disease risk in many studies. In one trial that included more than 6,000 women who were observed for nearly 17 years, those who ate fresh fruit every day had reduced mortality from heart disease. In a study on diet and blood pressure, Dr. Tom Vogt of the Center for Health Research in Portland, Oregon, found that when patients ate more fruits and vegetables—4 to 5 half-cup servings each day—and reduced dietary fat to 25 percent of daily calories, average blood pressure dropped as much as in studies where drugs for high blood pressure were used.

Whole grains, such as brown rice and millet, along with oats, oat bran, and most beans, provide soluble fiber. Try flax seed or oat bran sprinkled on cereal or low-fat yogurt.

Fish is the most healthy meat for those with risk factors for heart disease. Eating fish three to four times a week, or taking about 4 grams of fish oil a day, has been shown to help reduce blood clotting and triglycerides.

Nuts are a good source of protein and unsaturated oils. In the Iowa Women's Health Study of more than 40,000 menopausal women, a reduced risk of coronary heart disease was linked to nut consumption. Women who ate nuts five times a week cut their risk in half.

Red wine has been the subject of much recent research. The findings sound good if you like drinking wine, but the issue is far from settled. Some studies show a protective effect with only red wine, others with any alcohol, and some show an increased risk of heart attacks with red-wine consumption. What *is* certain is that purple grape juice and many fruits and vegetables have the same protective properties as red wine, and consuming more alcohol than one drink a day is probably not healthy.

Green tea has been shown to have a positive effect on serum cholesterol, triglycerides, and blood pressure. Green tea is also lower in caffeine than coffee, cola, or black tea. If you're trying to quit caffeine entirely, tablets and pills of green-tea extract are available. Unfortunately, nearly all green-tea research has been performed on men.

> ## FISH OIL OR FISH STORY?
>
> The omega-3 fatty acids found in fish and fish oils protect the heart and blood vessels. Fish-oil supplementation, on the other hand, is still not completely proven to help prevent heart disease, although some studies report positive effects. If you don't like fish, try adding foods that contain linolenic acid to the diet. This fatty acid is the precursor to omega-3; flax seeds and flaxseed oil are good sources.

Healthy Fats

It's easy to see why fat is so popular. It gives food a pleasing texture and satisfies a natural craving. Fat contains lots of calories, so it is a high-energy food. Even a healthy diet should include some fat—and it's certainly easier to stay on one that does.

But what's the difference between fat that's saturated and fat that isn't? And what about monounsaturated and polyunsaturated fats?

These terms about fat refer to its chemical structure and how many hydrogen atoms the fat molecule is carrying. If it is carrying as much hydrogen as it can, it is referred to as a saturated fat. These are the fats found in red meats, eggs, dairy products, and some vegetable oils, such as palm and coconut oils. Saturated fats can increase how much cholesterol is circulating in the bloodstream, leading to the clogging of arteries. Polyunsaturated fats, found in corn, cottonseed, safflower, soybean, sunflower, fish oils, and some margarine, are less damaging.

Hands down, our favorite fat is olive oil, which contains a mixture of saturated and monounsaturated fats. Olive oil may increase good HDL cholesterol while maintaining or lowering LDL, decreasing the risk of developing coronary artery disease. In addition, it may protect capillary walls by making them stronger and less permeable. Olive oil also may help regulate cholesterol by increasing bile production.

Beware of hydrogenated oils, whose molecular structure contains additional hydrogen atoms to keep the fat solid at room temperature. Hydrogenation creates harmful byproducts called trans-fatty acids. Margarine, which also contains hydrogenated oils, can be worse for your heart than the butter it replaces. The same goes for shortening, all-vegetable or not. Read food labels, and you'll see how common hydrogenated oils and fats have become.

CHOCOLATE: GOOD NEWS, BAD NEWS

The good news about chocolate is that a 1996 study suggests that its phenolic flavonoid compounds can help reduce LDL cholesterol by 75 percent, up to twice as much as red wine. A cup of hot chocolate—that's 2 tablespoons of cocoa—contains 146 mg of the protective compounds. A 1½-gram piece of milk chocolate, or 205 mg, is roughly equal to a 5-ounce glass of red wine.

Now for the bad news. The saturated fats in chocolate, mostly from palm-kernel oil or hydrogenated fats, can negate all the benefits from the flavonoids. And then, of course, there's the sugar and calories—a problem if you're trying to help your heart by losing weight.

Dietary Supplements

The evidence is not all in on whether supplements improve cardiovascular health. A review of studies performed over the last ten to fifteen years shows contradictions, so many physicians do not recommend most supplements. The exceptions are vitamin E and, usually, vitamin C. Even conservative medical researchers say that the evidence is fairly good that vitamin E helps prevent heart disease; it's also cheap and has few side effects.

Vitamin E may inhibit LDL oxidation, slow plaque formation, and reduce the risk of blood clotting. A study of more than 87,000 female nurses showed that vitamin E takes effect only after it is taken for two to eight years. Then the incidence of heart attack and stroke is reduced by 40 percent.

DINING OUT WISELY

Most restaurant foods have no labels and no indication of how much saturated fat a dish contains. Here are a few dining tips we have learned after years of trying to eat healthy despite hectic travel schedules.

Eat your veggies. Most chefs and cooks are willing to use low-fat methods, such as steaming, to make vegetable dishes. If a dish includes oil, your server should be willing to find out what kind. If the dish comes out bland, add tamari, soy sauce, or a squeeze of lemon.

The seafood diet. Salmon, red snapper, and halibut are healthy for the heart. Ask if you can get your fish broiled or poached without added sauces or oil, or with lemon instead of sauce.

Season with care. Ask your server for no MSG and no added salt. You can carry a shaker bottle of powdered sea vegetables such as wakame or nori, or vitamin C crystals, to give foods zing.

Try tubers. Baked potatoes are a good fiber source; add a little olive oil, herbs, or black pepper.

Heart-healthy desserts. In two words, fresh fruit—if you can get it without ice cream or cream sauce. Some restaurants offer non-fat yogurt.

Substitute soy. More restaurants have soy or veggie burgers these days, or offer dishes made with tofu or tempeh. Even in smaller cities, Chinese restaurants usually offer at least one tofu entree.

Better than butter. When the server brings the bread basket, ask for a small dish of olive oil for dipping.

Fiber, over easy. Instead of the fried foods most restaurants offer for breakfast, we ask for plain oatmeal and whole wheat toast, unbuttered. Some establishments offer fruit or nuts to put on the cereal.

Say *olé!* to avocados. Although high in fat, these staples of Mexican food are actually *good* for you; they can reduce total cholesterol and LDL cholesterol without lowering HDL cholesterol.

Speaking of Mexican food . . . Watch out for those chips. Corn, potato, and other types of fried chips are high in fat, not to mention all that salt. Ask if you can get baked chips or a stack of plain tortillas to go with your salsa or guacamole.

Vitamin C has also been found to be beneficial to heart disease patients in some cases. Vitamin C may transform vitamin E in the system to its active form and keep it working longer. It may also improve the health of blood vessels. In one study of 1,025 women and 835 men, the concentrations of vitamin C in the blood corresponded to an increase of "good" HDL in women, although not in men. When doctors recommend vitamins E and C, the usual doses are at least 1,000 mg of C and 400 IU of E.

Many of the B vitamins such as folic acid, B12, B6, and/or betaine hydrochloride can have a protective effect on the heart and cardiovascular system. In one large fourteen-year study, women with the highest folic-acid intakes had one-third fewer heart attacks than the women with the lowest intakes. Those who took vitamin B6 had a 6-percent lower risk for every milligram per day in their diets.

Some research has been done with two other supplements—coenzyme Q10 and vitamin D. In a study of 115 patients with high blood pressure, coenzyme Q10 supplementation resulted in lower blood pressure readings for 80 percent of subjects. CoQ10, as it is often called, has also been shown to have some benefits in mitral valve prolapse. Vitamin D deficiency and the resulting osteoporosis are seen in many people who have congestive heart failure.

Herbal Healing

Herbs have a long and revered history for preventing and reducing cardiovascular disease. The best-known heart herbs in Western herbalism are hawthorn and garlic. Women can benefit from these heart herbs beginning in their 40s, whether or not they have a family history of heart disease. Those with existing heart disease should consult a trained herbalist. Here are the major herbs for protecting and healing the heart and cardiovascular system, by category. We encourage you to experiment with one or two from each category, or blend several depending on your needs. Recipes follow the descriptions.

Heart Tonics

These herbs increase heart-muscle strength by improving the flow of nutrition and blood through the heart muscle and by balancing heart-cell metabolism.

BECOME A FIBER FAN

If you're eating a healthy diet, you may think you are getting enough fiber. But you may also benefit from a special fiber supplement. Taking a combination of flax seed, guar gum, and pectin that contains just five grams of fiber twice daily lowered cholesterol by 10 percent in one study.

Hawthorn. The leaves, flowers, and fruits of this plant are wonderful for strengthening and protecting the cardiovascular system, particularly the heart. Hawthorn is used to treat palpitations, angina, and hypertension. Studies show that the herb's combination of antioxidant compounds brings more blood into the heart itself while steadying the heartbeat, helping to lower blood pressure, and preventing clotting. A number of clinical trials show that hawthorn may help relieve symptoms of congestive heart failure.

Hawthorn can be taken as a tea, tincture, or standardized extract. Historically, the fruits or "berries" of hawthorn have been used, but new research has found that a combination of flowers and leaves makes an even more potent tonic. We recommend that any formula for heart disease include up to half hawthorn. This herb increases the potency of digitalis, so do not use these two remedies together unless your doctor advises it.

Night-blooming cereus. While you may not think of cacti when you think of medicine, this one makes an excellent cardiotonic and mild stimulant that strengthens and regulates the heartbeat. The extract is used for heart palpitations, angina pectoris, heart problems associated with tobacco use (such as congestive heart failure), and emphysema. Large doses of cereus tincture (more than 3 or 4 droppersful, 3 times per day) can lead to symptoms such as gastric irritation and heart irregularity, although this is rare.

Reishi. Traditional Chinese physicians believe that this mushroom imparts strength to the heart and other internal organs when taken regularly. If stress and insomnia are factors in your life, reishi will be a good addition to a heart formula. Drink 2 or 3 cups daily of reishi tea, or make a soup stock by shredding a medium-sized mushroom and simmering it in 2 quarts of water for an hour. Standardized extracts are available in liquid form, capsules, or tablets. We prefer red reishi extract.

Motherwort. This herb does double duty: For women, it benefits both the cardiovascular system and female organs. It strengthens the heart, allays palpitations, and regulates high blood pressure. Take one cup of a strong tea or 3 to 4 droppersful of the tincture morning and evening.

Blood Movers

Blood movers help the heart do its job by preventing stagnation of blood and vital energy in the heart muscle itself. Hawthorn and motherwort, previously described, are blood movers, as are the following herbs.

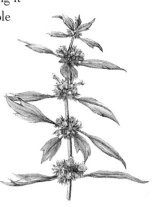

Motherwort

Ginkgo. Researchers are currently studying the leaves of this ancient Chinese tree, trying to pin down how it helps increase blood flow to the brain, peripheral arteries, and heart. Ginkgo's antioxidant properties make it a fine heart tonic as well. Numerous clinical trials have been performed with standardized ginkgo extract in the last fifteen years. More than 10 million prescriptions for it were written in 1989 in Germany and France.

Ginkgo not only improves circulation, it protects blood vessels, preventing abnormal leaking from tiny arteries. Some research suggests that ginkgo may reduce the risk of abnormal clotting—a major factor in heart attacks and stroke. In one study, 20 volunteers whose blood showed an increased tendency to form clots took 240 mg of ginkgo extract daily. Their blood thickness and clotting tendency was significantly reduced. A review of controlled trials performed on ginkgo over the last fifteen years found that about 75 percent of the elderly patients with artery blockage studied could walk further without pain.

Tinctures of ginkgo are not as potent as a standardized extract but are fine for prevention and as a daily tonic. The standardized extracts are available in pills or capsules.

Dan shen. Chinese red-sage root, or dan shen, is probably the best-known herb in Traditional Chinese Medicine for relieving blood stagnation and easing pain. The herb seems to have a mild cholesterol-lowering effect as well. Dan shen can be found whole in some herb shops or in tinctures in natural products stores.

Cholesterol Busters

Garlic. This aromatic herb is not only antibacterial, but has been shown to reduce cholesterol and exert a protective effect on the heart and blood vessels. Odor-controlled garlic supplements are available.

One review of 16 studies, including a total of 952 volunteer subjects, shows that although many of the trials were not well-designed, patients taking garlic experienced an average reduction of total cholesterol of 12 percent compared to those taking a placebo. One month of supplementation was required for full benefits. The authors of the review suggest a dose of 10 to 20 grams per day of fresh garlic or standardized fresh garlic perles, or at least 600 mg a day of dried garlic.

Artichoke leaf. Artichoke leaf-juice or extracts show good cholesterol-lowering effects in several human trials and are available in liquid, capsule, and tablet formulas. This herb and other bile-movers, such as wormwood, mugwort, and dandelion leaf, help improve blood health and fat digestion.

Cassia. This herb, *Cassia obtusifolia* or *C. tora*, also known as *jue ming zi*, is often used in China to treat people with mild or moderately elevated cholesterol levels. Effects are often felt within two weeks. Use about 2/3 ounce prepared as a decoction daily, drinking one cup both morning and evening. If using a powdered extract, take three 00-size capsules each morning and evening. Reduce the dose by one-half if your stools become loose; the herb is also prescribed as a laxative.

Hawthorn. This herb, discussed previously, also helps lower cholesterol levels.

Aromatherapy

A number of fragrances can help you relax, focus, and lower your blood pressure. Citrus fruits, ylang ylang, and marjoram contain essential oils that aid relaxation. For best results, incorporate the oils into a relaxing, blood-pressure-reducing massage or bath.

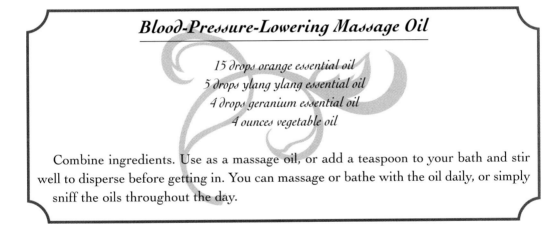

Blood-Pressure-Lowering Massage Oil

15 drops orange essential oil
5 drops ylang ylang essential oil
4 drops geranium essential oil
4 ounces vegetable oil

Combine ingredients. Use as a massage oil, or add a teaspoon to your bath and stir well to disperse before getting in. You can massage or bathe with the oil daily, or simply sniff the oils throughout the day.

SPECIAL SECTION ON VARICOSE VEINS

*T*he veins that run through our bodies help keep all tissues healthy. These flexible, delicate tubes carry spent blood back to the lungs for a refill of oxygen. The heart can pump this blood through the arteries, but it relies on muscle contractions to send it back through the veins. Thus the legs must move great volumes of blood upward to the heart. A series of valves stops the blood from falling back down into the legs, but its sheer weight, along with other factors, can produce faulty valves. Then the backflow of blood that results stretches out the veins, especially if they are already weakened by poor circulatory health.

Bulging, blue varicose veins appear most often on the legs. You are more likely to develop varicose veins if you sit or stand for long periods, so changing position and exercise help prevent them. Anything that constricts blood flow through the pelvic area can also be a cause—including being overweight, pregnant, or constipated, or wearing skin-tight pants or a girdle.

Nearly half the U.S. population has varicose veins; women are four times more likely than men to develop them. This is especially so during pregnancy. Varicose veins tend to run in families. If you have hemorrhoids—a specific type of varicose vein—you may have the conditions that cause varicose veins to develop in your legs.

Symptoms of varicose veins vary. They can make your legs tired, achy, and hot; some women don't feel them at all. Small, very superficial varicose veins, called spider veins, rarely produce symptoms. Larger varicose veins near the surface of the leg are unattractive but pose little risk.

Varicose veins deep in the leg, however, can cause serious trouble. When the leg's valves are insufficient, blood pools in the veins. As the veins become weaker, fluids and electrolytes can leak through the porous walls. Eventually, the varicose vein can burst and create slow-healing ulcers just under the skin. Clots may form, causing thrombophlebitis and increasing the risk of clots moving to the brain, heart, or lungs.

What a Doctor Will Do

Physicians consider varicose veins incurable but can perform surgery to remove the worst ones. There aren't many problems associated with this procedure, but after surgery, other weakened veins may break as they take on the extra blood load. Since bypass surgery uses the two main veins that run up the leg for grafts onto the coronary artery, physicians often prefer not to remove these veins in case they are needed in the future.

Another treatment, sclerotherapy, involves injecting a salt solution into the vein. It makes a clot that pinches off the vein, damaging and destroying it. Compression bandages are then wrapped around the leg from the toes up to the injection site and left in place for at least three weeks. There are few complications, but women must stop taking oral contraceptives for at least six weeks before and afterwards, since the pills encourage clotting.

Natural Healing

Dietary Changes

For healthy veins, eat a diet containing fiber-rich foods such as beans, vegetables, fruits, and whole grains. Try buckwheat—it not only has plenty of fiber but is loaded with the healthy flavonoid rutin, which can help improve the strength of blood-vessel walls. You can also drink a tea made from buckwheat leaves. During a three-month study of seventy-seven people at the Humboldt University in Berlin, buckwheat tea helped about half who drank it. The femoral vein, a major vein in the upper part of the legs, got smaller, and there was less permeability and leakage in the capillaries.

Other flavonoid-rich substances found in food are anthocyanidins. These colorants give bilberries, blueberries, purple grapes, and many other fruits and vegetables their deep coloring. Anthocyanidins protect blood-vessel walls and prevent leakage. They also increase intracellular vitamin C and collagen, making the connective tissue that supports blood vessels stronger. Anthocyanidins are now available in pill form. Proanthocyanidins (or OPCs), derived from either grape seed or pine bark, have similar properties.

Herbal Healing

To discourage blood clots, make cayenne, garlic, onions, and ginger plentiful in your diet. These herbs also improve the general health of veins. If you don't like to eat these herbs, they are available as supplements. Bromelain, derived from pineapple, has the same ability and can also be taken as a supplement. It is used in some hospitals to help prevent other veins from breaking after surgery. Take at least 500 mg of bromelain twice a day between meals.

One of the best ways to stop varicose veins from getting any worse is to improve their tone by making your blood vessels stronger and less porous and by tightening the elastic fibers in their walls, improving their flexibility and increasing blood flow. "Venotonics," as European doctors describe them, include some of the same herbs that have gained fame for treating heart problems—hawthorn, ginkgo, and gotu kola, among others. Horsechestnut and butcher's broom both encourage the movement of blood and prevent vessel leakage. Many formulas combine butcher's broom with vitamin C and the flavonoid hesperidin. Gotu kola strengthens connective tissue and the integrity of the protective sheath around the veins.

Several double-blind studies have shown the effectiveness of horse chestnut in treating varicose veins while relieving the uncomfortable itching and pain. In one three-month study, horse chestnut extract improved varicose veins as much as taking a diuretic and wearing compression stockings combined. Out of 240 people, both methods produced close to a 25-percent reduction in the amount of blood in the lower leg. Horse chestnut can be toxic in large doses, however, so use with care. We have also found horse chestnut cream highly effective for some people.

Aromatherapy

The essential oils of chamomile, palmarosa, myrtle, frankincense, and cypress reduce enlarged veins, ease inflammation, and lessen pain. These essential oils can be added to massage oils and gently rubbed on the veins. When massaging the legs, use gentle strokes; these veins are already fragile.

If the skin breaks over varicose veins or hemorrhoids, apply a clean cloth soaked in a solution of ten drops of essential oil and half a cup of water. Carrot seed essential oil helps the inflammation associated with enlarged veins, though it can be difficult to find.

Tea for Varicose Veins

2 teaspoons dried hawthorn berry and flower
2 teaspoons dried gotu kola leaf
1 quart water

Heat water to boiling; remove from heat and steep herbs for 5 minutes. Drink two cups a day. These herbs can also be taken as pills or tinctures.

CHAPTER 16

OSTEOPOROSIS

One of the most lasting gifts we can offer our daughters is an active lifestyle that builds strong bones while they are young.

Most women know an elderly person, perhaps a grandmother, who led a fairly normal life until an accidental fall and hip fracture. Suddenly, a vital individual became an invalid. Sometimes older people seem to be shrinking, not from weight loss, but in height. Occasionally an older woman gradually becomes hunched over with a "dowager's hump."

These problems are caused by a bone disorder known as osteoporosis, a gradual decrease of bone density that leads to weakness in bone structure. Far from being an inert structural element, bone is a dynamic living tissue that is constantly changing.

Throughout a woman's life, calcium is added to and subtracted from her bones in a continuous process. Ideally, this process is kept in equilibrium by a number of hormones and other substances. Cells called osteoclasts absorb old bone tissue, while cells known as osteoblasts lay down new bone tissue. Ideally, this process maintains the bones in maximum strength and health.

With age, bones lose an excessive amount of protein and minerals; the osteoblasts cannot keep up with this loss. Over time, this can lead to osteoporosis, literally "porous bone," a condition of low bone mass and density. Women with osteoporosis are susceptible to broken bones and fractures, including severely painful fractures of the vertebrae.

Annually, as many as 40 percent of American Caucasian women over the age of 50 may suffer from osteoporosis and many experience at least one fracture as a result. The treatment of these 1.5 million fractures costs about $10 billion each year; the cost will likely reach $240 billion within 50 years as the number of aging women increases. Of 100 women 65 years old, 1 to 2 will have an osteoporosis-related fracture; 6 to 10 of every 100 women age 75 will have one. Fractures of the spine are most common, but any weak bone can break.

Hip fractures are dangerously debilitating, and recovery is often long and uncertain. Those who survive often face limita-

Horsetail

tions in activity and loss of independence. Hip fracture also increases the possibility of death within five years by about 20 percent.

Only in the last few decades has it come to light that bone building and maintenance in youth and early adulthood play a crucial role in preventing osteoporosis. During childhood, a girl's body builds bone. Peak bone mass—the strongest the bones will ever be—is usually achieved during the 20s. After about age 35, bone loss begins to exceed new-bone buildup.

The period of most rapid bone loss is the first five to nine years past menopause. As estrogen production decreases in the first two years, one to 2 percent bone loss occurs. After ten years, the annual rate of bone loss drops to 0.5 percent. If a woman—even one with significant risk factors—takes early measures to build bone mass, she can minimize the effects of aging on her bones.

Who Gets Osteoporosis?

Certain conditions can lead to osteoporosis in young women, and about 20 percent of cases occur in men, but dangerous osteoporosis leading to fractures is most commonly associated with estrogen deficiency in postmenopausal women. Caucasian and Asian women are at higher risk than Hispanic or African-American women. So are small-statured, thin-boned women, regardless of race. Genetic heritage plays an important role; osteoporosis in your mother or grandmother means your risk is higher.

Some drugs contribute to loss of bone mass and density. The most damaging, because of the frequency of their use, are the glucocorticoids or corticosteroids such as cortisone, which are taken for inflammatory diseases. Women who take these drugs for long periods for such ailments as rheumatoid arthritis, asthma, or chronic obstructive lung disease tend to have higher rates of osteoporosis. Use of the anticoagulant Heparin, anticonvulsive drugs such as Dilantin, and thyroid supplements are also associated with increased rates of bone loss.

A number of diseases spur development of osteoporosis, including Cushing's disease, diabetes, anorexia nervosa, bulimia, Crohn's disease, irritable bowel syndrome, hyperthyroidism, hyperparathyroidism, liver disease, multiple myeloma, and kidney failure. Some diseases affect bone growth through hormonal imbalance; others cause poor absorption of nutrients or interfere with the nourishment of tissues.

WHAT A DOCTOR WILL DO

A visit to the doctor should include a complete physical exam with a patient history designed to assess the patient's risk of osteoporosis.

Unfortunately, the first clear symptom of osteoporosis is often a broken bone; by then, serious bone loss has already occurred. Early clinical diagnosis of osteoporosis is difficult.

The most accurate way to diagnose osteoporosis is by bone-density measurements, but this is expensive and not readily available. Instead, a physician will usually request tests for blood calcium, phosphorus, estrogen, and other hormones. Various X-rays may also be requested. Although X-ray will indicate bone loss, it is not sensitive enough to diagnose early osteoporosis. Computed tomography or CT scan is slightly more sensitive than X-ray. Only the women at greatest risk for osteoporosis should have a bone density test.

Bone mass is measured in a variety of ways, depending on the type of bone being scanned. Measuring two bones, for instance a hip and a vertebra, provides a fairly accurate picture of bone strength. Bone density is often measured in grams per centimeter, and experts disagree about the point at which risk begins. One study reports that women with a bone density of greater than 1.0 gm/cm signals a normal risk for bone fracture, 0.8 to 1.0 gm/cm signals a moderate risk, and less than 0.8 gm/cm signals high risk.

Drug Treatments

About half of medical doctors believe that for postmenopausal patients facing osteoporosis, estrogen-replacement therapy is the best treatment to slow the loss of bone mass, increase bone-mineral density, and avoid fractures.

Estrogen-replacement therapy, however, carries increased risk of uterine and possibly breast cancer. The longer estrogen is used, the greater the risk may be. Generally, hormone replacement is begun when menopausal symptoms first appear. It usually continues for ten years or more.

A new class of drugs called selective estrogen-receptor modulators (SERMs) may offer some benefits without the risks of estrogen itself. Raloxifene, currently the only medication in this category marketed to prevent osteoporosis, has estrogen-like effects on bone tissue but does not

RISK FACTORS AT A GLANCE

If you are a woman between the ages of 40 and 60, you may benefit from a check of your bone density, especially if you also have one or more of the following factors.

Family history of fractures, osteoporosis, or diabetes

Low estrogen levels

Thin build or history of being underweight

No use of estrogen or birth-control pills

Early menopause

Hysterectomy before menopause, even if the ovaries are retained

No children

Regular, moderate-to-heavy use of alcohol

Sedentary lifestyle

Smoking, current or in the past

Long-term use of steroids or thyroid medications

stimulate breast or uterine tissue. Like estrogen, it also helps prevent heart disease.

Aminobisphosphonates such as alendronate (Fosamax) and etidronate (Didronel) are new drugs prescribed for osteoporosis or the risk of it. They inhibit the activity of osteoclasts, decreasing bone resorption. When taken over time, these drugs decrease the rate of bone loss. The drugs' major drawback is irritation of the stomach lining and esophagus; if taken with anti-inflammatories such as aspirin, they can cause ulcers.

The amount of estrogen in the blood is important. Estrogen acts by increasing bone growth, in part by increasing the release of the thyroid hormone calcitonin. This substance acts to inhibit osteoclasts, the bone-resorbing cells. It also acts by taking calcium from the blood to deposit in bone. Estrogen also stimulates the bone-building cells, or osteoblasts, to promote bone growth. That is why postmenopausal women are more prone to osteoporosis than younger women. Doctors sometimes prescribe injections of calcitonin itself (Miacalcin) to increase bone density and mass; but the drug must be combined with calcium to prevent bone

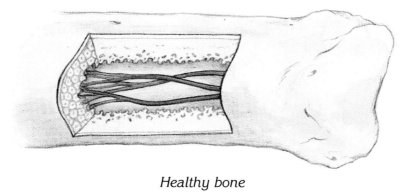

Healthy bone

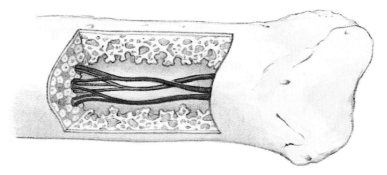

Bone with osteoporosis

loss. For either estrogen or calcitonin to function, the woman taking them must also be getting adequate calcium and vitamin D.

Fluoride salts are sometimes used to prevent bone loss. Intermittent fluoride may be used in addition to other treatments.

NATURAL HEALING

The primary predictor of osteoporosis is heredity, but increasing the amount of bone mass early in life through diet and exercise decreases the impact of osteoporosis later. Having eaten poorly and failed to exercise when you were young does not necessarily doom you to a fragile old age. At any time in your life, you can take important steps to optimize bone strength and prevent falls. Osteoporosis is a lifestyle illness; improving one's diet and exercise patterns is helpful at any age.

Healthy Habits

If Aunt Mary falls and breaks her hip, you could blame her post-menopausal age, the thin build she inherited, or the fact that she smoked until she was 60. You could blame society for making athletic pursuits unfashionable when she was a teenager. You could fault the high-blood-pressure medication that made her dizzy, her brightly waxed and slippery floor, or the low coffee table that tripped her. Or you could examine her slowly decreasing exercise level and diminishing balance and coordination.

While Aunt Mary is recovering from the fall — or before you or someone in your life has one — some immediate changes can reduce risks.

Most hip fractures are the direct result of a fall. Those at risk for fractures, and those who love the folks at risk, should fall-proof the home. Eliminate slippery floors, loose throw rugs, clutter, trailing electrical cords, and low furniture. Install good lighting, sturdy stairway railings, and handrails and non-slip footing in showers and bathtubs. Bring essential supplies within reach and make sure the elderly do not carry cumbersome loads. When advanced osteoporosis and debility raise the chances of fracture from a fall, protective hip pads may be in order.

Many medications, particularly those for high blood pressure, can cause balance problems or decreased alertness. Changing the drug or the schedule of use may be helpful.

Most hip fractures are the direct result of a fall. Women at risk for fractures, and those who love the women at risk, should fall-proof the home.

Diseases that are not associated with lowered bone density but that cause impaired balance, unsteadiness, dizziness, or decreased vision also can lead to a fall. Parkinson's disease, inner-ear disorders, seizure disorders, and other neurological diseases are some of the most obvious. Muscle disease or cardiovascular disease also may predispose a woman to falling.

Smoking weakens bones and causes other health problems. Smokers face a risk of hip fracture 40 to 50 percent higher than nonsmokers. A smoking cessation program, even after a lifetime of smoking, can offer some defense against serious injuries from falls.

Smokers face a risk of hip fracture that is 40 to 50 percent higher than nonsmokers.

Exercise: Both Prevention and Cure

The best preventive measure against osteoporosis—for *all* women of *all* ages—is exercise. In young adulthood, it builds bone density. In old age, it not only prevents bone loss but helps women retain the coordination and balance that may help them avoid a fall or minimize injury when one occurs.

Strengthening exercises such as weight-training are as important as calcium for strong bones, and they can be started at any age. Exercise improves agility, balance, strength, and mood. Fear of falling causes many older women to reduce their activities, so gaining strength and balance and improving mood can be a real benefit.

A study of bone growth in children finds that lack of physical activity is a major factor in low bone-mineral density. Another study of preadolescent gymnasts found greater hip-bone density compared to that of a control group of healthy, nonathletic girls.

Encouraging girls to engage in physical activity is one of the greatest gifts we can give, whether they are team players or loners by nature. If your daughter seems disinterested in the competitive sports that tend to dominate school athletic programs, seek out other ways for her to get the exercise that will be crucial to her bones in years to come.

For older women, exercise—especially walking—is helpful. Bones need the pressure of weight upon them to lay down new bone tissue. Engaging in weight-bearing exercise for thirty minutes daily, or for up to an hour several times weekly, slows bone loss. In a study of thirty-six women who ate similar diets, eighteen walked for slightly less than an hour four days a week. The other half of the group continued their sedentary ways. Half of the women in each group drank a high-calcium drink every day. After one year, the sedentary women lost an average of

7 percent of spine bone, while the walkers increased spine bone by half a percent. Those who used the calcium drink gained about another 2 percent of hip-bone density.

Weight training is effective even for women in their 80s who have very little strength. When done several times per week, it tones muscles, ligaments, and even bone. In one double-blind, controlled study, thirty-nine postmenopausal women performed five exercises with weights two days a week. After one year, the density of the femoral neck bone and lumbar spine increased 1 percent, and muscle strength and balance also improved. The bone density of women in a control group that did not exercise fell 2.5 percent; strength and balance deteriorated.

While weight-bearing exercise is the most effective, it's not practical for some. A recent study found that isometric exercise contracting and releasing isolated muscles consistently builds both muscles and bones. Women who find it physically or emotionally difficult to walk, run, or go to the gym can exercise this way.

DON'T RETIRE, PERSPIRE

William Evans of the U.S. Department of Agriculture and Human Nutrition Research Center on Aging at Tufts University is adamant that what we need as we age is not more rest, but more exercise, especially weight-training. He calls the decline of strength and vitality normally associated with aging "heading into the disability zone" (Evans, 1992).

Here are Dr. Evans's tips for weight training.

Lift enough weight so that your muscles are fatigued after eight or nine repetitions. On most weight machines, this is about twenty pounds for a healthy woman of 65.

If you don't have access to a gym, fill a gallon milk container with water. It will weigh about eight pounds—a good starting weight for arm exercises.

Big rubber bands for resistance exercises are inexpensive and available at sporting goods stores.

Don't begin lifting too quickly or hold your breath while doing so; lift slowly and smoothly.

Warm up and cool down. The goal is muscle fatigue, not pain.

Start by lifting two or three days a week, with rest days in between to give your muscles a chance to repair.

Dietary Changes

Calcium, the key element of bone, is essential in maintaining your body's structural health. Unfortunately, calcium, as well as other components that help the body use it, are typically deficient in diets of the elderly in the United States. Adding high-calcium foods and eliminating those that remove calcium or prevent its absorption is a good start to a program for bone health.

CALCIUM SUPPLEMENT DOSAGES	
Birth to 6 months	600 mg
1 to 5 years	800 mg
6 to 10 years	800–1200 mg
11 to 24 years	1200–1500 mg
25 to 50 years	1000 mg
Pregnant, lactating	1200 mg
Postmenopausal, with estrogen replacement	1000 mg
Postmenopausal, without estrogen replacement	1500 mg

(Source: National Institute of Health, 1994)

A varied diet containing lots of high-quality vegetables, grains, and dairy products will usually provide ample calcium. If your diet is not optimum and not easily changed, doctors and herbalists alike recommend nutritional supplements, especially vitamin D, calcium, and magnesium. Vitamin D promotes calcium absorption. About thirty minutes of sun provides your body with up to 400 IU or more of vitamin D. Consuming adequate levels of magnesium and vitamin D, along with getting enough physical activity, can help maintain optimum bone density throughout life.

The Dairy Dilemma

Dairy products rate high on any list of calcium-rich foods. Yet a relatively large number of women with osteoporosis do not properly digest milk. This condition, known as lactose intolerance, occurs when lactase, the enzyme that digests lactose, is deficient. Within a group of women with osteoporosis, 35 percent were lactase deficient, compared to only one out of thirty-one women in a control group.

If you cannot digest milk products, prefer nondairy sources of calcium, or simply want more calcium in your diet, many foods can supply it. Sardines, salmon, figs, and dark green, leafy vegetables such as collard and turnip greens contain high amounts of calcium. Green leafy vegetables are also slightly bitter, which promotes assimilation of nutrients, and they contain good amounts of magnesium and other important minerals. Eating foods such as these with lemon juice or apple cider vinegar increases their acidity, giving assimilation a second boost.

Digestion is not the only problem with commercial dairy products. Commercial dairies often do whatever is necessary to increase production while reducing costs. Antibiotics, steroids, and hormones are often added to the cows' diet to increase production; current U.S. laws do not require consumer notification when these products are used. Organic dairy products are becoming more widely available.

Protein and Other Nutrients

The level of protein in the diet can affect osteoporosis. Protein is made up of amino acids, most of which are necessary for the body to build strong bone from calcium. Researchers have known for some time that women with protein deficiency, or whose diet does not contain all the essential amino acids, especially L-lysine, have problems using calcium. In an animal study where L-lysine and L-arginine were added to a rat's

DIETARY SOURCES OF CALCIUM

Food	Serving Size		Calcium (mg)
Parmesan cheese, grated	1	ounce	390
Collard greens, cooked from frozen, chopped	1	cup	357
Sardines, canned in oil	8	medium	354
Rhubarb, cooked, sugar added	1	cup	348
Yogurt (lowfat)	8	ounces	345
Milk, skim	1	cup	303
Blackstrap molasses	2	tablespoons	274
Figs, dried	10	figs	269
Turnip greens	1	cup	267
Spinach, cooked from raw	1	cup	245
Cheddar cheese	1	ounce	211
Creamed cottage cheese	1	cup	211
Kale	1	cup	206
Broccoli, cooked, drained	1	spear, medium	205
Mustard greens	1	cup	193
Salmon, canned (pink)	3	ounces	167
Dandelion greens	1	cup	147
Bok choy	1	cup	116
Tofu	1/2	cup cubed	108
Dried whole sesame seeds	1	tablespoon	88
Almonds	12	nuts	39

Source: Pennington, 1994

drinking water, the supplements doubled the uptake of calcium into the bones. Greater absorption of calcium also occurred in the intestine. Don't overdo protein consumption, however. Excess protein—more than 70 or so grams a day—actually decreases calcium in the body.

For fighting osteoporosis, vegetarian protein is often preferred over animal protein as a dietary mainstay. In comparative studies, vegetarians consistently have higher bone densities than meat-eaters. Why? Protein sources such as soy may offer a more easily accessible form of calcium. Further, the green leafy vegetables that are abundant in a *good* vegetarian diet are full of magnesium to help the assimilation of calcium.

Soy products and many other beans also contain natural estrogenic compounds called phytoestrogens. These compounds may be the reason why women living in Asian countries have a much lower rate of hip fractures than women in Western countries. Asian women also eat more seaweed and fish—both foods rich in minerals.

In one study of soy products, researchers examined 80 post-menopausal women who ate 1/2 cup tofu every day. This amount is the botanical equivalent of taking 20 mg of conjugated estrogens from the hormone-replacement drug Premarin. Early results found that bone-loss rates went down. Phytoestrogens also help protect the heart and vascular system and may help prevent some kinds of cancers.

Foods to Avoid

Some foods decrease bone density or interfere with the absorption of calcium. Calcium loss in the urine can be traced to excess consumption of alcohol, caffeine, protein, sodium, and the phosphoric acid used in many soft drinks. In a three-year study of 980 postmenopausal women, aged 50 to 98 years, a significant association was made between a lifetime of consuming caffeinated coffee and loss of bone density in hips and spines. Interestingly, coffee drinkers who also drank a glass of milk daily didn't show the same loss.

Soft drinks are of great concern since many people, especially children, consume large amounts of them, often as a replacement for milk or water. Cola drinks are especially worrisome. The phosphoric acid and caffeine they contain can leach calcium from the bones and weaken them. One study of 76 girls and 51 boys found a strong association between cola consumption and bone fractures in the girls.

To Imbibe or Not?

Finally, alcohol use increases the danger of falls, but very moderate use may actually decrease the risk of osteoporosis by increasing estrogen levels. In a 5-year study of 128 women, researchers found that estrogen levels increased with 3 drinks a week. After about 6 drinks a week, however, estrogen levels stabilized. Moderation is always the key.

Dietary Supplements

Studies proving that calcium supplementation prevents bone loss are legion. One four-year study tracked eighty-four women, ages 54 to 74, who were more than ten years past menopause. The women took an average of 2 grams of calcium a day for the duration of the study, while the control group took an average of 1 gram a day. The high-calcium group showed no bone loss at the hip and ankle, while the women in the control group did lose bone. Neither group lost bone in the spine.

A study from the University of Auckland in New Zealand found that when women who were at least three years past menopause took a gram of calcium per day, they halved their expected bone loss.

Many physicians suggest 1.5 grams calcium daily for postmenopausal women. The Food and Drug Administration recommends about the

FOODS TO AVOID
Coffee and other caffeinated drinks
An overall high-fat diet
Refined sugar and foods and drinks that contain it
Daily consumption of alcohol
Very low or very high protein intake

BONE HEALTH AND TRADITIONAL CHINESE MEDICINE

In Traditional Chinese Medicine, the kidneys are thought to be responsible for bone strength. While weak kidneys may be inherited, habits such as coffee drinking, excessive sexual activity, lack of rest, and a poor diet can seriously deplete their strength.

When the kidneys are depleted, the areas of the body they govern will show signs of weakness—a sore lower back and knees, hearing problems, premature gray hair, and weak bones. Though Western medicine usually views these symptoms as unrelated, traditional Chinese physicians view them as a connected syndrome. A recent Western study, however, shows a correlation between osteoporosis and premature graying; subjects with premature graying, but no other risk factors for osteoporosis, were more than four times as likely to show bone loss as subjects without premature graying.

Traditional Chinese Medicine treats osteoporosis with kidney-building herbs. Japanese teasel root *(Dipsacus asper)*, for example, is used to strengthen the bones and heal fractures. The herb's Chinese name, *xu duan*, literally means "restore what is broken." Another bone-mending herb is the rhizome of a fern, *Drynaria fortunei*. Its Chinese name, *gu sui bu*, translates to "mender of shattered bones."

same: 1 to 2 grams (1,000 to 2,000 mg) a day to reduce the risk of osteoporosis. The price of calcium supplementation is relatively cheap: about fifty cents a day.

The Limits of Calcium Supplements

Clearly, calcium helps prevent osteoporosis, and in some cases may reverse bone loss in postmenopausal women. But there are limits to its effectiveness. Some forms of calcium are more effective than others for some people; some supplements have risks or side effects. Unfortunately for women between the ages of 30 and menopause, the ability of calcium supplements to build bone or prevent bone loss remains unproven. Nonetheless, some physicians recommend up to 1 gram of calcium per day for premenopausal women. Calcium supplementation may be contraindicated if you have reason to be concerned about kidney stones, hyperparathyroidism, sarcoidosis, or kidney failure. And too much calcium can cause problems, including calcification of soft tissue.

Calcium carbonate, found in many supplements including Tums, requires plenty of stomach acid to break it down. Studies show, however, that about 40 percent of menopausal women have deficient stomach acid, and can only absorb about 4 percent of this type of calcium. In fact, a recent study of 241 individuals found that the use of Tums as a calcium supplement was associated with a higher risk of upper-arm fracture.

Calcium citrate is very absorbable, even for those with low stomach acid, because it *is* an acid. With sufficient stomach acid, calcium gluconate, lactate, malate, and aspartate are also absorbable forms. On the other hand, the increasingly popular calcium hydroxyapatite, derived from bone meal, is poorly absorbed. Plus, oyster shell, dolomite, and particularly bone meal can contain large amounts of lead. Even those with normal amounts of stomach acid absorb only about 22 percent of this type of calcium. One solution is to take an ionized form of calcium, such as calcium citrate, because it can be more easily absorbed than calcium salts.

> ## HOW TO TAKE CALCIUM
>
> It is best to take calcium supplements morning and evening with meals to maximize absorption; your digestive tract can only absorb so much calcium at once. If you are taking iron supplements as well, take them separately, because calcium can block the absorption of iron.

Other Supplements

Several other nutrients are essential for building and maintaining strong bones. These include vitamin D, magnesium, phosphorus, and, to a lesser extent, copper.

Vitamin D helps the gastrointestinal tract absorb calcium, and the relationships among the intake of calcium and vitamin D and bone strength have been the subject of many recent studies. Among the findings are the need for extra vitamin D when taking calcium supplements; one study suggests that women taking 500 mg of calcium daily should take at least four times that amount of vitamin D daily. Another study of women with osteoporosis who suffered recent hip fractures found that many have lower vitamin D levels than other women. The researchers concluded that vitamin D's relationship to bone strength is so important that assuring adequate levels of vitamin D for the elderly should be adopted as a public health objective.

The usual dose of vitamin D is 400 to 800 IU, but those who are past menopause and have either high cholesterol or heart disease should consult a nutritionist or other qualified health-care practitioner to determine appropriate dosage. Vitamin D can increase both overall cholesterol and LDL cholesterol—the so-called "bad" cholesterol.

Nearly as important as calcium is magnesium. People who develop osteoporosis are more likely to be deficient in magnesium than others. We agree with nutritionists who recommend that patients take twice as much magnesium as calcium.

Also important, though of less proven benefit to bone density and osteoporosis prevention, are the trace minerals manganese, potassium, copper, boron, fluoride, strontium, and silicon, as well as vitamins C, B6, B12, K, and folic acid. Vitamin K helps bones retain calcium and may play a role in preventing osteoporosis. This may be one reason why vegetarian women who eat plenty of vitamin K in green, leafy vegetables have less osteoporosis.

Boron slows the excretion of calcium through the urine. It also assists the conversion of vitamin D in the kidneys and the bone-preserving actions of estrogen. Vitamin C is necessary in the formation of collagen. Potassium reduces calcium excretion from the body.

TESTING YOUR CALCIUM SUPPLEMENT AT HOME

If your calcium supplement is in tablet form, here's a quick test to see how rapidly it breaks down and is assimilated in your digestive tract. Drop a tablet into a small glass of vinegar and stir several times. If the tablet mostly dissolves within 30 minutes, chances are you will absorb a significant amount of its calcium.

Herbal Healing

Herbs that we recommend to help maintain strong bones include those that are mineral-rich and promote good assimilation. Herbs called adaptogens, which support adrenal function and reduce the impact of stress, are also helpful; we recommend eleuthero and American ginseng.

Mineral-Rich Herbs

Good herbal sources of calcium are dandelion greens, watercress, and parsley. Some calcium is also found in nettles, red clover, alfalfa, and horsetail. Of this collection, the most widely recommended herbs for strengthening bone, hair, skin, and nails are nettle leaf and horsetail. Herbalists call nettles nature's vitamin pill because they contain calcium, magnesium, phosphorus, and good-quality protein. Horsetail is nature's source of silica, traditionally thought to help the body assimilate calcium. Standardized horsetail products (certified to contain a certain amount of silicic acid, the natural, organic form of silica) are available in capsule or tablet form.

Strong Bones Broth

This broth can be added to soups or stews or used instead of water to cook rice. It includes ginger to increase mineral assimilation and eleuthero to support the adrenal glands.

2 cups horsetail
2 cups nettle leaf
1 cup dandelion, watercress, or parsley greens or any combination
1/4 cup chopped fresh ginger root
1/8 cup eleuthero (Siberian ginseng)
8 cups water

Simmer the herbs for 45 minutes in water in a stainless steel pot. Strain the broth and press as much liquid from the herbs as possible; discard herbs. Drink 1 cup broth morning and evening, before meals, or use in cooking. Store in refrigerator for up to 4 days.

RESOURCE DIRECTORY

OTHER BOOKS BY KATHI KEVILLE

Herbs for Chronic Fatigue. 1998. New Canaan, CT: Keats.

Herbs: An Illustrated Encyclopedia. 1994. New York: Friedman/ Fairfax

Pocket Guide to Aromatherapy. 1996. Freedom, CA: The Crossing Press.

Herbs for Health and Healing. 1996. Emmaus, PA: Rodale Press, Inc.

Aromatherapy, A Complete Guide to the Healing Art (with M. Green.) 1995. Freedom, CA: The Crossing Press.

OTHER BOOKS BY CHRISTOPHER HOBBS

Handmade Medicines. 1998. Loveland, CO: Botanica/Interweave Press.

Stress and Natural Healing. 1997. Loveland, CO: Botanica/Interweave Press.

St. John's Wort, The Mood Enhancing Herb. 1997. Loveland, CO: Botanica/Interweave Press.

The Ginsengs. 1996. Santa Cruz, CA: Botanica Press.

Handbook for Herbal Healing. 1994.

Santa Cruz, CA: Botanica Press.

Valerian, The Relaxing and Sleep Herb. 1993. Santa Cruz, CA: Botanica Press.

Foundations of Health. 1992. Santa Cruz: Botanica Press.

Vitex, The Women's Herb. 1990. Santa Cruz: Botanica Press.

Echinacea, The Immune Herb. 1990. Santa Cruz: Botanica Press.

Natural Liver Therapy. 1986. Santa Cruz: Botanica Press.

RECOMMENDED READING

Women's Health

Conney, S. 1994. *The Menopause Industry: How the Medical Establishment Exploits Women.* Alameda, CA: Hunter House.

Crawford, Amanda McQuade. 1997. *Herbal Remedies for Women.* Rocklin, CA: Prima Publishing.

Crawford, Amanda McQuade. 1996. *The Herbal Menopause Book.* Freedom, CA: The Crossing Press.

Gladstar, Rosemary. 1993. *Herbal Healing for Women.* New York: Simon & Schuster.

Hudson, Tori. 1992. *Gynecology and Naturopathic Medicine.* Aloha, OR: TK Publications.

Love, Susan. 1990. *Dr. Susan Love's Breast Book*. Reading, MA: Addison-Wesley.

Lowdog, T. 1995. *A Natural Approach to Women's Health*. Albuquerque, NM: Hound Dog Productions. (2-part video)

Northrup, C. 1994. *Women's Bodies, Women's Wisdom*. New York: Bantam.

Ojeda, L. 1995. *Menopause without Medicine*. Alameda, CA: Hunter House.

Seaman, B. and G. Seaman. 1997. *Women and the Crisis in Sex Hormones*. New York: Bantam Books.

Soule, D. 1995. *The Roots of Healing: A Woman's Book of Herbs*. New York: Citadel Press.

Weed, S. 1996. *Breast Cancer? Breast Health*. Woodstock: Ash Tree Publishing.

Weed, S. 1985. *Herbal for the Childbearing Years*. Woodstock, NY: Ash Tree Press.

Other Topics

Beinfield, H. and E. Korngold. 1991. *Between Heaven and Earth, A Guide to Chinese Medicine*. New York: Ballantine.

Eskin, B. A. 1994. *The Menopause: Comprehensive Management*. New York: McGraw-Hill, Inc.

Felter, H. W. and J. U. Lloyd, eds. 1983. (1898). *King's American Dispensatory*. Portland, OR: Eclectic Medical Publications.

Flint, M., F. Kronenberg, and U. Wulf (Eds.). 1990. Multidisciplinary Perspectives on Menopause. *Annals of the New York Academy of Sciences*, Vol. 592.

McGuffin, M. et al. 1997. *Botanical Safety Handbook*. Boca Raton, FL: CRC Press.

HERB ASSOCIATIONS

American Botanical Council
6200 Manor Road
Austin, TX 78723
800-373-7105
abc@herbalgram.org

American Herb Association
PO Box 1673
Nevada City, CA 95959
530-265-9552

American Herb Products Association
4733 Bethesda Avenue
Bethesda, MD 20814

Herb Research Foundation
1007 Pearl St.
Boulder, CO 80302

National Association for Holistic Aromatherapy
836 Hanley Industrial Court
St. Louis, MO 63144

United Plant Savers
PO Box 420
Barre, VT 05649

ASSOCIATIONS AND
SUPPORT GROUPS

AIDS Action Committee
131 Clarendon St.
Boston, MA 02116
617-437-6200

Bosom Buddy Club
1057 Columbia Pl.
Boulder, CO 80303
303-494-8252
(women's resource guide)

Cancer Control Society
2043 N. Berendo St.
Los Angeles, CA 90027
213-663-7801

**Cancer Treatment Centers of
America** at Midwestern
Regional Medical Center
2520 Elisha Ave.
Zion, IL 60099
800-577-1255
www.cancercenter.com

Endometriosis Association
8585 N. 76th Pl.
Milwaukee, WI 53223
800-992-ENDO
800-426-2END (Canada)

**Endometriosis Treatment
Program**
St. Charles Medical Center
2500 NE Neff Rd.

Bend, OR 97701
800-486-6368

Asha Resource Center
PO Box 13827
Research Triangle Park, NC
27709
919-361-8488
800-230-6039
(national herpes hotline)

**The North American
Menopause Society**
Post Office Box 94527
Cleveland, OH 44101
216-844-8748
Fax 216- 844-8708
e-mail: nams@apk.net

**Midwives Alliance of North
America**
PO Box 175
Newton, KS 67114
316-283-4543

**National Osteoporosis
Foundation, Dept MQ**
PO Box 96616
Washington, DC 20077-7456

**National Women's Health
Network**
Washington, DC 20004
202-628-7814
(informational packets)

HERB PERIODICALS
**American Herb Association
Newsletter**
PO Box 1673
Nevada City, CA 95959

Herbalgram
6200 Manor Road
Austin, TX 78723

Herbs for Health
201 East Fourth St.
Loveland, CO 80537-5655

Medical Herbalism
PO Box 20512
Boulder, CO 80308

Meno Times
1108 Irwin St.
San Rafael, CA 94901
(newsletter)

Menopause News
2074 Union St.
San Francisco, CA 94123
800-241-MENO
www.well.com/(ews
(newsletter)

Women's Health Connection
PO Box 6338
Madison, WI 53716
800-366-6632
(newsletter)

WESTERN HERBS AND PRODUCTS

Avena Botanicals
219 Mill St.
Rockport, ME 04856
207-594-0694
tinctures, oils, salves

Frontier Herb Co-op
PO Box 299

Norway, IA 53218
800-669-3275
bulk herbs and products, certified organics, free catalog

Green Terrestrial
328 Lake Avenue
Greenwich, CT 06830
203-862-8690
tinctures, herbal products

Herb Pharm
Box 116
Williams, OR 97544
800-348-4372
tinctures, salves

Herbalist & Alchemist
PO Box 553
Broadway, NJ 08808
908-689-9020
tinctures, Western and Chinese herbs

Jean's Greens
119 Sulphur Spring Rd
Newport, NY 13416
888-845-8327
herbs, oils, containers, teas

Pacific Botanicals
4350 Fish Hatchery Rd.
Grants Pass, OR 97527
541-479-7777
certified organic, fresh and dried herbs by the pound

Rainbow Light
207 McPherson
Santa Cruz, CA 95060

800-635-1233
800-227-0555 (in California)
tinctures, caplets, vitamins

Way of Life
1210 41st Ave.
Capitola, CA 95010
408-464-4113
clay, castor oil, dried herbs, oils

Wise Woman Herbals
PO Box 279
Creswell, OR 97426
541-895-5172
800-532-5219
tinctures, glycerites, oils, salves

CHINESE HERBS AND PRODUCTS

Mayway Corporation
1338 Mandela Parkway
Oakland, CA 94607
800-262-9929
liquid extracts, Chinese herbs

Tashi/Min Tong Herbs
5221 Central Ave., Suite 105
Oakland, CA 9460
800-538-1333

ESSENTIAL OILS

Oak Valley
PO Box 2482
Nevada City, CA 95959
(catalog $1)

Original Swiss Aromatics
Pacific Institute of Aroma
Therapy
PO Box 6723
San Rafael, CA 94903
415-479-3979

Simplers Botanical, Co.
PO Box 2534
Sebastapol, CA 95473
800-652-7646
organic extracts, essential oils

TINCTURE SUPPLIES

McCormick Distilling
Westin, MO 64098
800 825-0377

Aaper Alcohol Company
PO Box 339
Shelbyville KY 40065

HEALTH INFORMATION ONLINE

National Library of Medicine
(800) 638-8480.
http://www.nlm.nih.gov

REFERENCES

CHAPTER 1: WOMEN'S HEALTH

Bagchi, D. et al. 1997. Oxygen free-radical scavenging abilities of vitamins C and E, and a grape-seed proanthocyanidin extract *in vitro*. *Research Communications in Molecular Pathology and Pharmacology* February 95(2):179–89.

Blumenthal, M. et al (Eds.). 1996. *Commission E Herbal Monographs*. Austin, TX: American Botanical Council.

Bone, M. E. et al. 1990. Ginger root—a new antiemetic. The effect of ginger root on postoperative nausea and vomiting after major gynaecological surgery. *Anaesthesia* Aug. 45(8):669–71.

Chang, H. and P. P. But. 1986. *Pharmacology and Applications of Chinese* Materia Medica. Singapore: World Scientific.

Coeugniet, E. G. and R. Kuhnast. 1986. Recurrent candidiasis: Adjutant immunnotherapy with different formulations of Echinacin. *Therapiewoche* 36:3352–58.

Cohen et al. 1997. Social ties and susceptibility to the common cold. *JAMA* 277(24): 1940–44.

Ellingwood, F. 1983. (1898). *American Materia Medica, Therapeutics and Pharmacognosy*. Portland, OR: Eclectic Medical Publications.

Felter, H. W. and J. U. Lloyd. 1876. *King's American Dispensatory*. Cincinnati: The Ohio Valley Co.

Foster, S. and J. Duke. 1990. *A Field Guide to Medicinal Plants: Eastern and Central North America*. Boston: Houghton-Mifflin Co.

Gunn, J. C. 1875. *Gunn's New Family Physician*. Cincinnati: Wilstach, Baldwin, and Co.

Hobbs, C. *The Ginsengs, A User's Guide*. Santa Cruz, CA: Botanica Press.

Hobbs, C. 1986. *Usnea: The Herbal Antibiotic*. Santa Cruz, CA: Botanica Press.

Hobbs, C. 1990. *Vitex, The Women's Herb*. Santa Cruz: Botanica Press.

Hobbs, C. and S. Brown. 1997. *Saw Palmetto: The Herb for Prostate Health*. Loveland, CO: Botanica/Interweave Press.

Hobbs, C. and S. Foster. 1990. Hawthorn, a literature review. *Herbalgram* 22: 19–33.

Keville, K. and M. Green. 1995. *Aromatherapy: A Complete Guide to the Healing Art*. Freedom, CA: The Crossing Press.

Moore, M. 1979. *Medicinal Plants of the Mountain West*. Santa Fe: The Museum of New Mexico Press.

Newall, C. A. et al. 1996. *Herbal Medicines: A Guide for Health-Care Professionals*. London: The Pharmaceutical Press.

United Press International. 1997. Exercise slows aging, researchers say. November 7.

United Press International. 1997. Study says most Canadians are overweight. December 4.

Van Den Broucke, C. O. 1983. The therapeutic value of *Thymus* species. *Fitoterapia* 4:171–74.

Verma, S. 1988. WHO marks 50th anniversary with warning for future. Reuters News Service, April 6.

Weiss, R. F. 1986. *Herbal Medicine*. Gothenburg, Sweden: AB Arcanum.

Weissbuch, B. K. 1998. Personal communication.

Wren, R. C. 1988. *New Cyclopaedia of Botanical Drugs and Preparations*. Essex, England: C. W. Daniel Co. Ltd.

CHAPTER 2: WOMEN'S HORMONES

Allen, L. H. 1994. Nutritional supplementation for the pregnant woman. *Obstetrics and Gynecology* 37:587–95.

Brigden, M. L. 1993. Iron deficiency anemia: Every case is instructive. *Postgraduate Medicine* 93:181–92.

CHAPTER 3: ANEMIA

Dorgan, J. F. et al. 1997. Relationship of serum dehydroepiandrosterone (DHEA), DHEA sulfate, and 5-androstene-3 beta, 17 beta-diol to risk of breast cancer in post-menopausal women. *Cancer Epidemiology Biomarkers.* In *Prevention* Mar. 6(3):177–81.

Duke, James. 1998. Personal communication.

Eskeland, B. et al. 1997. Iron supplementation in pregnancy: Is less enough? *Acta Obstetricia et Gynecologica Scandinavica* 76(9): 822–8.

Freire, W. B. 1997. Strategies of the Pan-American Health Organization/World Health Organization for the control of iron deficiency in Latin America. *Nutrition Reviews* 55(6): 183–8.

Gibbons, W. E. 1998. Experience with a novel vaginal progesterone preparation in a donor oocyte program. *Fertility and Sterility* 69(1):96–101.

Gleerup, A. et al. 1995. Iron absorption from the whole diet: Comparison of the effect of two different distributions of daily calcium intake. *American Journal of Clinical Nutrition* 61: 997–1004.

Hannigan, B. M. 1994. Diet and immune function. *British Journal of Biomedical Sciences* 51:252–59.

Heersche, J. N. et al. 1998. The decrease in bone mass associated with aging and menopause. *Journal of Prosthetic Dentistry* Jan. 79(1):14–16.

Hunt, J. R. et al. Effect of vitamin C on iron absorption by women with low iron stores. *American Journal of Clincial Nutrition* 59:1381–85.

Khaw, K. R. 1996. Gender and cardio-vascular risk. *Journal of Human Hypertension* June 10(6):403–07.

Looker, A. et al. 1997. Prevalence of iron deficiency in the United States. *Journal of the American Medical Association* March 26, 973–76.

Nelson, M. et al. 1994. Iron-deficiency anemia and physical performance in adolescent girls from different ethnic backgrounds. *British Journal of Nutrition* 72:427–433.

Pennington, J. A. T. 1994. *Bowes & Church's Food Values of Portions Commonly Used* (16th ed.). Philadelphia: J. B. Lippincott Co.

Weinberg, E. D. 1993. The iron-with-holding defense system. *American Society for Microbiology News* 59:559–62.

Weinberg, E. D. and G. Weinberg. 1995. The role of iron in infection. *Current Opinion in Infectious Diseases* 8:164–69.

Werbach, M. R. 1988. *Nutritional Influences on Illness.* Tarzana, CA: Third Line Press.

Woolf, S. H. 1993. Routine iron supplementation during pregnancy: Policy statement. *JAMA* 270(23):2846–47.

Yokoi, K. et al. 1994. Iron and zinc nutriture of premenopausal women: Associations of diet with serum ferritin and plasma-zinc disappearance and of serum ferritin with plasma zinc and plasma-zinc disappearance. *Journal of Laboratory and Clinical Medicine* 124:852–61.

CHAPTER 4: MOOD DISORDERS

American Psychiatric Association. 1994. *Diagnostic and Statistical Manual of Mental Disorders* (4th ed.). Washington, DC: American Psychiatric Association.

Braverman, E. R. 1987. *The Healing Nutrients Within.* New Canaan, CT: Keats Publishing.

Barrett, J. E. et al. 1988. The prevalence of psychiatric disorders in a primary care practice. *Archives of General Psychiatry* 45(12):1100.

Horner, J. 1995. Psychological issues. In Carr, P. L. et al. (Eds.). *The Medical Care of Women.* Philadelphia: W. B. Saunders.

Miller, J. B. 1983. The construction of anger in women and men. Work in Progress 83:01. Wellesley, MA: Stone Center Working Papers Series.

Werbach, M. R. 1988. *Nutritional Influences on Illness.* Tarzana, CA: Third Line Press.

CHAPTER 5: MENSTRUATION

Amman, W. 1982. Amenorrea. *Zeitschrift Alligeneinmed* 58:228–31.

Charlton, A. and D. While. 1996. Smoking and menstrual problems in 16-year-olds. *J. R. Soc. Med.* 89(4):193–5.

Harlow, S. D. and M. Park. 1996. A longitudinal study of risk factors for the occurrence, duration, and severity of menstrual cramps in a cohort of college women. *British Journal of Obstetrics and Gynaecology* Nov. 103(11):1134–42.

Lithgow, D. M. and W. M. Politzer. 1977. Vitamin A in the treatment of menorrhagia. *S. Afr. Med. J.* 12;51(7):191–3.

Yaginuma, T. 1982. Effect of traditional herbal medicine on serum testosterone levels and its induction of regular ovulation in hyperandrogenic and oligomenorrheic women. *Nippon Sanka Fujinka Gakkai Zasshi* 34(7):939–44.

CHAPTER 6: PMS

Abraham, G. E. 1983. Nutritional factors in the etiology of the PMS. *Journal of Reproductive Medicine* 28:446–64.

Baker, E. R. et al. 1995. Efficacy of progesterone vaginal suppositories in alleviation of nervous symptoms in patients with premenstrual syndrome. *Journal of Assisted Reproduction and Genetics* 12(3):205–9.

Bennett, D. R. et al (Eds.). 1991. *Drug Evaluations Annual, 1991.* Milwaukee: American Medical Association.

Dalton, K. 1977. *The Premenstrual Syndrome and Progesterone Therapy.*

London: William Heinermann Medical Books, Ltd.

Freeman, E. et al. 1995. A double-blind trial of oral progesterone, alprazolam, and placebo in the treatment of severe premenstrual syndrome. *JAMA* 274(1):51–57.

Gardner, K. and D. Sanders. 1993. Premenstrual syndrome. In McPherson, A. (Ed.). *Women's Problems in General Practice.* New York: Oxford University Press.

Goei, G. S. et al. 1982. Dietary patterns of patients with premenstrual tension. *J. Applied Nutr.* 34(1):4–11.

Johnson, E. A. et al. 1985. Efficacy of feverfew on prophylactic treatment of migraine. *British Medical Journal* 291:569–73.

Jones, D. V. 1987. Influence of dietary fat on self-reported menstrual symptoms. *Physiological Behavior* 40(4):483–87.

Keltner, N. L. and D. G. Folks. 1993. *Psychotropic Drugs.* St. Louis: Mosby.

London, R. S. et al. 1983. The effect of alpha-tocopherol on premenstrual symptomatology: A double-blind trial. *J. Amer. Col. Nutr.* 2:115–122.

Mortola, J. F. 1995. Premenstrual syndrome. In Carr, P. L. et al (Eds.). *The Medical Care of Women.* Philadelphia: W. B. Saunders Company.

Rossignol, A. M. 1985. Caffeine–containing beverages and premenstrual syndrome in young women. *American Journal of Public Health* 75(11):1335–37.

Thys-Jacobs, S. 1994. Vitamin D and calcium in menstrual migraine. *Headache* 34(9):544–546.

CHAPTER 7: ENDOMETRIOSIS

Barnard, N. 1994. Natural progesterone: Is estrogen the wrong hormone? *Good Medicine* Spring, 11–13.

Christensen, B. et al. 1995. Endometriosis—diagnosis and therapy. Results of a current survey of 6,700 gynecologists. *Geburtshilfe*

Frauenheilk 55(12):674–79.

Falcone, T. et al. 1996. Endometriosis: Medical and surgical intervention. *Current Opinions in Obstetrics and Gynecology* 8(3):178–83.

Gerhard, I. et al. 1992. Auricular acupuncture in the treatment of female infertility. *Gynecology and Endocrinology* Sept., 6(3):171–81.

Gleicher, N. 1994. The role of humoral immunity in endometriosis. *ACTA Obstetricia et Gynecologica Scandinavica* Suppl 159:15–17.

Grodstein, F. et al. 1994. Infertility in women and moderate alcohol use. *American Journal of Public Health* Sept. 84(9):1429–32.

Laufer, M. R. et al. 1997. Prevalence of endometriosis in adolescent girls with chronic pelvic pain not responding to conventional therapy. *Journal of Pediatric and Adolescent Gynecology* Nov. 10(4):199–202.

Marcoux, S. et al. 1997. Laparoscopic surgery in infertile women with minimal or mild endometriosis. *New England Journal of Medicine* July 24, 337(4):217–22.

Pouly, J. L. et al. 1996. Laparoscopic treatment of symptomatic endometriosis. *Human Reproduction* Nov. 11, Suppl 3:67–88.

Rier, S. E. et al. 1995. Immunoresponsiveness in endometriosis: Implications of estrogenic toxicants. *Environmental Health Perspective* 103 Suppl 7:151–56.

Saidi, M. H. et al. 1996. Complications of major operative laparoscopy: A review of 452 cases. *Journal of Reproductive Medicine* July, 41(7):471–76.

Sutton, C. J. et al. 1997. Follow-up report on a randomized controlled trial of laser laparoscopy in the treatment of pelvic pain associated with minimal to moderate endometriosis. *Fertility and Sterility* Dec. 68(6):1070–74.

Tsenov, D. 1996. The effect of acupuncture in dysmenorrhea. *Akusherstsvo i Ginekologiya (Sofiia)* 35(3):24–25.

Chapter 8: Fibroids and Cysts

Apesteguia, L. et al. 1997. Nonpalpable, well-defined, probably benign breast nodules: Management by fine-needle aspiration biopsy and long-interval follow-up mammography. *European Radiology* 7(8):1235–9.

Brooks, S. E. 1995. Uterine leiomyomas. In Carr, P. L. et al (Eds.), *The Medical Care of Women.* Philadelphia: W. B. Saunders Co.

Harrison-Woolrych, M. and R. Robinson. 1995. Fibroid growth in response to high-dose progestogen. *Fertility & Sterility* 64(1):191–2.

Healy, D. L. et al. 1992. The role of GnRH agonists in the treatment of uterine fibroids. *British Journal of Obstetrics & Gynaecology* 99 (suppl 7):23–6.

Sifton, D. W. (Ed.). 1994. *The PDR Family Guide to Women's Health and Prescription Drugs.* Montvale, NJ: Medical Economics.

Smith, R. P. 1997. *Gynecology in Primary Care.* Baltimore: Williams & Wilkins.

Stolz, W. and Pfutzenreuter, N. 1997. Treatment of uterine leiomyoma with depot leuprorelin acetate (Enantone-Gyn monthly depot). Effect on leiomyoma volume and operability. German Leuprorelin Study Group. *Zentralbl Gynakol* 119(10):468–75.

Chapter 9: Vaginal Infections

Bensky, D. and A. Gamble. 1993. *Chinese Herbal Medicine* Materia Medica. Seattle: Eastland Press.

Berkow, R. et al (Eds.). 1992. *The Merck Manual* (16th ed.). Rahway, NJ: Merck & Co. Inc.

Carr, P. L. 1995. Infectious disease in women. In Carr, P. L. et al (Eds.), *The Medical Care of Women.* Philadelphia: W. B. Saunders Co.

CHAPTER 10: URINARY TRACT INFECTIONS

Hamilton-Miller, J. M. T. 1994. Cranberry juice, bacteriuria, and pyuria. *JAMA* 272(8):588.

Harrison, W. O. et al. 1974. A prospective evaluation of recurrent urinary tract infection in women. *Clin. Res.* 22:125A.

Kuzminski, L. N. 1996. Cranberry juice and urinary tract infections: Is there a beneficial relationship? *Nutrition Reviews* (II):S87–S90.

Schacht, M. J. 1993. Recurrent urinary tract infections. In Knaus, J. V. and J. H. Isaacs (Eds.). *Office Gynecology: Advanced Management Concepts.* Berlin: Springer-Verlag.

Sergio, W. et al. 1988. Zinc salts that may be effective against the AIDS virus, HIV. *Medical Hypothesis* 26:251–3.

Sulis, C. 1995. Infectious disease in pregnancy. In Carr, P. L. et al. *The Medical Care of Women.* Philadelphia: W. B. Saunders Co.

CHAPTER 11: SEXUALLY TRANSMITTED DISEASES

Apisariyakulm, A. 1990. Zinc monoglycerolate is effective against oral herpetic sores. *Medical Journal of Australia* 152:54.

Becker, T. M. et al. 1994. Sexually transmitted diseases and other risk factors for cervical dysplasia among southwestern Hispanic and non-Hispanic white women. *JAMA* 271(15):1181–8.

Braverman, E. R. 1987. *The Healing Nutrients Within.* New Canaan, CT: Keats Publishing.

Hording, U. Prevalence of human papillomavirus types 11, 16 and 18 in cervical swabs. A study of 1,362 pregnant women. *European Journal of Obstetrics, Gynecology, and Reproductive Biology* 35(2–3):191–8.

Libman, H. 1995. Sexually transmitted diseases. In Carr, P. L. et al (Eds.).

The Medical Care of Women. Philadelphia: W. B. Saunders Co.

McCrone, E. L. 1995. Human immunodeficiency virus infection: Epidemiology, risk assessment, and testing. In Carr, P. L. et al (Eds.). *The Medical Care of Women.* Philadelphia: W. B. Saunders Co.

Sifton, D. W. (Ed.). 1994. *The PDR Family Guide to Women's Health and Prescription Drugs.* Montvale, NJ: Medical Economics.

Sulis, C. 1995. Infectious disease in pregnancy. In Carr, P. L. et al. *The Medical Care of Women.* Philadelphia: W. B. Saunders Co.

Tay, S. K. 1995. Genital oncogenic human papillomavirus infection: A short review on the mode of transmission. *Ann. Acad. Med. Singapore* 24(4):598–601.

CHAPTER 12: CERVICAL DYSPLASIA

Babbs, C. F. 1992. Oxidative radicals and ulcerative colitis. *Free Radical Biology and Medicine* 13:169–81.

Baldauf, J. J. et al. 1992. Role of herpes virus simplex and cytomegalovirus as cofactors of papillomavirus in dysplastic and cancerous lesions of the uterine cervix. *Chirurgie* 118(10):652–8.

Becker, T. M. 1994. Sexually transmitted diseases and other risk factors for cervical dysplasia among southwestern Hispanic and non-Hispanic white women. *JAMA* 271(15):1181–8.

Benmoura, D. et al. 1986. Cervical screening and surveillance of the cervix uteri before the age of 20. *J. Gynecol. Obstet. Biol. Reprod.* (Paris) 15(1):63–71.

Bosch, F. X. et al. 1997. Human papillomavirus and other risk factors for cervical cancer. *Biomed Pharmacother* 51(6–7): 268–75.

David, M. et al. 1993. Changes in cervix cytology in women with liver transplants treated with immunosuppressive therapy. *Zentralbl Gynakol* 115(8):362–5.

de Vet, H. C. et al. 1993. The role of sexual factors in the aetiology of cervical dysplasia. *Int. J. Epidemiol* 22(5):798–803.

de Vet, H. C. et al. 1994b. Risk factors for cervical dysplasia: Implications for prevention. *Public Health* 108(4):241–9.

Eduardo, C. E. et al. 1995. Papillomavirus in cervicovaginal smears of women infected with human immunodeficiency virus. *Revista Paulista de Medicina* 113(6):1009–11.

Engineer, A. D. and J. S. Misra. 1987. The role of routine outpatient cytological screening for early detection of carcinoma of the cervix in India. *Diagnostic Cytopathology* 3(1):30–4.

Grail, A. and M. Norval. Significance of smoking and detection of serum antibodies to cytomegalovirus in cervical dysplasia. *British Journal of Obstetrics and Gynaecology* 95(11):1103–10.

Ho, G. Y. et al. 1995. Persistent genital human papillomavirus infection as a risk factor for persistent cervical dysplasia [see comments]. *Journal of the National Cancer Institute* 87(18):1365–71.

Meekin, G. E. 1992. Prevalence of genital human papillomavirus infection in Wellington women. *Genitourinary Medicine* 68(4):228–32.

Miller, K. E. 1992. Evaluation and follow-up of abnormal Pap smears. *American Family Physician* 45(1):143–50.

Mitchell, M. F. et al. 1995. Chemoprevention trials and surrogate end-point biomarkers in the cervix. *Cancer* 76(10 Suppl):1956–77.

Moore, B. C. et al. 1995. Predictive factors from cold-knife conization for residual cervical intraepithelial neoplasia in subsequent hysterectomy. *American Journal of Obstetrics and Gynecology* 173(2):361–68.

Naumann, R. W. 1996. Treatment of cervical dysplasia with large loop excision of the transformation zone: Is endocervical curettage necessary? *Southern Medical Journal* 89(10):961–5.

New Zealand Contraception and Health Study Group. 1989. The prevalence of abnormal cervical cytology in a group of New Zealand women using contraception: A preliminary report. *New Zealand Medical Journal* 102(872):369–71.

Nishioka, K. et al. 1995. Polyamines as biomarkers of cervical intraepithelial neoplasia. *Journal of Cellular Biochemistry.* Supplement, 23:87–95.

Palan, P. R. 1991. Plasma levels of antioxidant beta-carotene and alpha-tocopherol in uterine cervix dysplasias and cancer. *Nutrition and Cancer* 15(1):13–20.

Shy, K. et al. 1989. Papanicolaou smear screening interval and risk of cervical cancer. *Obstet. Gynecol* 74:838–43.

Warren, D. L. and A. Duerr. HIV infection in nonpregnant women: A review of current knowledge. *Current Opinion in Obstetrics and Gynecology* 5(4):527–33.

Ziegler, R. G. 1996. Epidemiologic studies of vitamins and cancer of the lung, esophagus, and cervix. *Advances in Experimental Medicine and Biology* 206:11–26.

CHAPTER 14: MENOPAUSE

Carr, B. R. 1996. HRT management: The American experience. *European Journal of Obstetrics, Gynecology, and Reproductive Biology* 64 Suppl:S17–20.

Carter, B. F. and P. J. Fink. 1994. Psychiatric myths of the menopause. In *Menopause, Comprehensive Management* (3rd ed.). New York: McGraw-Hill.

Finkler, R. S. 1949. The effect of vitamin E in the menopause. *Journal of Clinical Endocrinology and Metabolism* 9:89–94.

Flint, M., F. Kronenberg, and U. Wulf (Eds.). 1990. Multidisciplinary perspectives on menopause. *Annals of the New York Academy of Sciences*, Vol. 592.

Hammer, M. 1990. Does physical exercise influence the frequency of postmenopausal hot flashes? *Acta Obstetrics and Gynecol Scandinavia* 69:409–12.

Kalogeraki, A. et al. 1996. Cigarette smoking and vaginal atrophy in postmenopausal women. *In Vivo* Nov.-Dec. 10(6):597–600.

Kaufert, P. and J. Syrotuik. 1981. Symptom reporting at the menopause. *In Social Science and Medicine. Part E, Medical Psychology* Aug.

Knight, D. and J. Eden. 1996. A review of the clinical effects of phytoestrogens. *Obstetrics & Gynecology* 87(5):897–904.

Kronenberg, F. 1990. Hot flashes: Epidemiology and physiology. *Annals of the New York Academy of Sciences* 592.

Lock, M. 1994. Menopause in cultural context. *Experimental Gerontology* 29(3,4):307–17.

McCoy, N. et al. 1985. Relationships among sexual behavior, hot flashes, and hormone levels in perimenopausal women. *Archives of Sexual Behavior* 14:385–88.

McKinley, S. M. and M. Jefferys. 1974. The menopausal syndrome. *British Journal of Preventive Social Medicine* 28:108:15.

McLaren, H. 1949. Vitamin E in the menopause. *British Medical Journal* 37:350.

Shute, E. 1937. Notes on menopause. *Journal of the Canadian Medical Association* 37:350.

Smith, R. P. 1997. *Gynecology in Primary Care.* Baltimore: Williams & Wilkins.

Subbiah, M. T. 1998. Mechanisms of cardioprotection by estrogens. *Proceedings of the Society for Experimental Biology and Medicine* 217(1):23–29.

Utian, W. 1997. Women view menopause as a new beginning. Reuters News Service, September 8.

Chapter 15: Heart Disease, including Varicose Veins

Abbott, R. D. et al. 1988. High density lipoprotein cholesterol, total cholesterol screening, and myocardial infarction: The Framingham Study. *Arteriosclerosis* 8:207.

Agren, J. J. et al. 1996. Fish diet, fish oil, and decosahexaenoic acid lower fasting and postprandial plasma lipid levels. *European Journal of Clinical Nutrition* 50:765–71.

American Health Foundation. 1995. Exploring the chemopreventive properties of tea. *Primary Care and Cancer: American Health Foundation Update* February. 15(2):30–31.

American Heart Association, 1997. Women underrate heart, stroke risks. Reuters News Service, New York, September 9.

Ayanian, J. Z. and A. M. Epstein. 1991. Differences in the use of procedures between women and men hospitalized for coronary heart disease. *New England Journal of Medicine* 325:221.

Bensky, D. and A. Gamble. 1993. *Chinese Herbal Medicine* Materia Medica. Seattle: Eastland Press.

Blumenthal, J. A. et al. 1997. Stress control lowers cardiac risk. *Archives of Internal Medicine* 157:2213–23.

Brown, M. et al. 1997. Improvement of insulin sensitivity by short-term exercise training in hypertensive African-American women. *Hypertension* Dec. 30(6):1549–53.

Carmena, R. et al. 1980. Olive oil dietary supplement. *Third International Congress on Biological Value of Olive Oil Report*, Crete, Greece.

Chae, C. et al. 1997. *Frequent Exercise Best for Heart.* Annual meeting, American Heart Association, Orlando, FL.

de Lorgeril, M. 1996. Control of bias in dietary trial to prevent coronary recurrence: The Lyon Diet Heart Study. *European Journal of Clinical Nutrition* 51:116–22.

Diehm, C. et al. 1996. Comparison of leg compression with chronic venous insufficiency. *The Lancet* 347:292–94.

Ernst, E. 1996. *Ginkgo biloba* in treatment of intermittent claudication: A systematic research based on controlled studies in the literature. *Fortschritte der Medizin* 20;114(8):85–87.

Harvard Mens Health Watch. 1998. Margarine, trans-fatty acids, and the heart: A promise not kept. Mar. 2(8):5–7.

Heart attack and peanuts. 1997. *Nutrition Week* 27(37):8.

Hoffman, R. M. and H. S. Garewal. 1995. Antioxidants and the prevention of coronary heart disease. *Archives of Internal Medicine* 155:241–46.

Hoogeveen, E. K. et al. 1978. Hyperhomocysteinemia is associated with a risk of cardiovascular disease, especially in noninsulin diabetes mellitus. *Arteriosclerosis, Thrombosis, and Vascular Biology* Jan. 18:133–381.

Ihme, I. et al, 1995. Leg edema protection from buckwheat herb tea in patients with chronic venous insufficiency. *European Journal of Clinical Pharmacology* 50:443–47.

Key, T. et al. 1996. Dietary habits and mortality in 11,000 vegetarians and health-conscious people: Results of a 17-year follow-up. *British Medical Journal* 313:775–79.

Kris-Etherton, P. and D. Krummel. 1993. Role of nutrition in the prevention and treatment of coronary heart disease in women. *Journal of the American Dietetic Association* 93:987–94.

Langsjoen, P. H. et al. 1993. Isolated diastolic dysfunction of the myocardium and its response to CoQ10 treatment. *Clinical Investigator* 71:S 140–S 144.

Lindberg, G. et al. 1998. Use of calcium channel blockers and risk of suicide: Ecological findings confirmed in population-based cohort. *British Medical Journal* 7:316 (7133): 741–45.

Malcolm, G. T. et al. 1997. Risk factors for atherosclerosis in young subjects: The PDAY study. Pathological determinants of atherosclerosis in youth. *Annals of the New York Academy of Sciences* May 28, 817:179–88.

Nehler, M. R. et al. 1997. Homocysteinemia as a risk factor for atherosclerosis: A review. *Cardiovascular Surgery* 5(6):559–67.

Pellegrini, N. et al. 1996. Effects of moderate consumption of red wine on platelet aggregation and haemostatic variables in healthy volunteers. *European Journal of Clinical Nutrition* 50:209–13.

Russell, R. M. 1997. Soy protein and nutrition. *JAMA* 277(23):1876–78.

Samman, S. 1997. Nutrition and therapeutics. *Current Opinion in Lipidology* 8:U47–U48.

Shane, E. 1997. Mass, vitamin D deficiency, and hyperparathyroidism in congestive heart failure. *American Journal of Medicine* 103:197–207.

Sifton, D. W. (Ed.). 1994. *The PDR Family Guide to Women's Health and Prescription Drugs.* Montvale, NJ: Medical Economics.

Silagy, C. and A. Neil. 1994. Garlic as a lipid lowering agent: A meta-analysis. *Journal of the Royal College of Physicians of London* 28(1):39–45.

Stampfer, M. et al. 1991. Postmenopausal estrogen therapy and cardiovascular disease: Ten-year follow-up from the Nurse's Health Study. Abstracted. *New England Journal of Medicine* 325:756.

Stavric, B. 1994. Role of chemopreventers in human diet. *Clinical Biochemistry* 7(5):319–32.

Vogt, T. 1997. A clinical trial of the effects of dietary patterns on blood pressure. *New England Journal of Medicine* 336:117–24.

Waterhouse, A. L. et al. 1996. Antioxidant chocolate. *The Lancet* Sept. 348:834.

Weihmayr, T. and E. Ernst. 1996. Therapeutic effectiveness of *Crataegus. Fortschritte der Medizin* 114(1–2):27–29.

Witte, S. et al. 1993. Improvement of hemorrheological parameters with *Ginkgo biloba* extracts. *Fortschritte der Medizin* 13:247–50.

Woolf-May, K. et al. 1997. Effects of an 18-week walking programme on cardiac function in previously sedentary or relatively inactive adults. *British Journal of Sports Medicine* 31:48–53.

Zoler, M. L. 1997. High folic acid intake lowers heart attack risk. *Family Practice News* August 1, 1997;1.

CHAPTER 16: OSTEOPOROSIS

Barrett-Connor, E. et al. 1994. Coffee-associated osteoporosis offset by daily milk consumption: The Rancho Bernardo study. *Journal of the American Medical Association* 271(4):280–83.

Bell, N. H. and R. H. Johnson. 1997. Bisphosphonates in the treatment of osteoporosis. *Endocrine* 6(2):203–06.

Binkley, N. C. and J. W. Suttie. Vitamin K nutrition and osteoporosis. *Journal of Nutrition* 125:1812–21.

Bourgoin, B. P. et al. 1993. Lead content in 70 brands of dietary calcium supplements. *American Journal of Public Health* 83:1155–60.

Bullock, C. 1995. Soybeans: An estrogen-replacement alternative? *Family Practice News* April 6, p. 11.

Carr, C. J. and E. F. Shangraw. 1987. Nutritional pharmaceutical aspects of calcium supplementation. *American Pharmacy* 27:49–57.

Coats, C. 1990. Negative effects of high protein diet. *Family Practice Recertification* 12(12):80–88.

Cooper, C. 1997. The crippling consequences of fractures and their impact on quality of life. *American Journal of Medicine* 103(2A):12S–19S.

Cumming, R. G. et al. 1997. Calcium intake and fracture risk: Results from the study of osteoporotic fractures. *American Journal of Epidemiology* 145(10):926–34.

Dawson-Hughes, B. 1997. Effect of calcium-vitamin D supplementation on bone density in men and women 65 years of age and older. *The New England Journal of Medicine* 337(10):670–76.

Devine, A. et al. 1997. A four-year follow-up study of the effects of calcium supplementation on bone density in elderly postmenopausal women. *Osteoporosis International* 7(1):23–28.

Dyson, K. et al. 1997. Gymnastic training and bone density in pre-adolescent females. *Medicine and Science in Sports and Exercise* 29(4):443–50.

Eaton-Evans, J. et al. 1996. Copper supplementation and the maintenance of bone-mineral density in middle-aged women. *The Journal of Trace Elements in Experimental Medicine* 9:84–87.

Farrerons, J. et al. 1997. Sodium fluoride treatment is a major protector against vertebral and nonvertebral fractures when compared with other common treatments of osteoporosis: A longitudinal, observational study. *Calcified Tissue International* 60(3):250–54.

Freund, K. M. 1995. Osteoporosis. In Carr, P. L. et al (Eds.). *The Medical Care of Women.* Philadelphia: W. B. Saunders Co.

Furst, M. D. 1993. Dietary L-lysine supplementation: A promising nutritional tool in the prophylaxis and treatment of osteoporosis. *Nutrition* 9(1):71–72.

Hathcock, J. N. 1997. Vitamins and minerals: Efficacy and safety. *American Journal of Clinical Nutrition* 66:427–37.

Heaney, R. 1993. Thinking straight about calcium. *New England Journal of Medicine* Feb. 18, 328(7):503–05.

Heikkinen, A. M. et al. 1997. Long-term vitamin D3 supplementation may have adverse effects on serum lipids during postmenopausal hormone replacement therapy. *Eur. J. Endocrinol* 37(5):495–502.

Hopper, J. L. and E. Seeman. 1994. The bone density of female twins discordant for tobacco use. *New England Journal of Medicine* 330:387.

Kanis, J. A. et al. 1994. Perspective: The diagnosis of osteoporosis. *Journal of Bone Mineral Research* 9:1137–41.

Kapetanos, G. et al. 1997. A double-blind study of intranasal calcitonin for established postmenopausal osteoporosis. *Acta Orthopaedica Scandinavica Supplementum* 275:108–11.

Lems, W. F. et al. 1997. Is addition of sodium fluoride to cyclical etidronate beneficial in the treatment of corticosteroid-induced osteoporosis? *Annals of Rheumatological Disease* 56(6):357–63.

Lindsay, R. 1995. The burden of osteoporosis: Cost. *American Journal of Medicine* 98(Suppl. 2A):2A–9S to 2A–11S.

Nelson, M. E. 1991. A 1-Y walking program and increased dietary calcium in postmenopausal women: Effects on bone. *American Journal of Clinical Nutrition* 53:1304–11.

Newcomer, A. D. et al. 1978. Lactase deficiency: Prevalence in osteoporosis. *Ann. Intern. Med.* 89(2):218–20.

Nieves, J. W. et al. 1998. Calcium potentiates the effect of estrogen and calcitonin on bone mass: Review and analysis. *American Journal of Clinical Nutrition* 67(1):18–24.

Orcel, P. 1997. Calcium and vitamin D in the prevention and treatment of osteoporosis. *Revue Du Rhumatisme* (English edition) 64(6 Suppl): 70S–74S.

Pfeiffer, N. 1992. Moderate drinking may cut osteoporosis. *Medical Tribune* July 23:3.

Quesada-Gomez, J. M. et al. 1996. Vitamin D insufficiency as a determinant of hip fracture. *Osteoporosis International* 3:S42–S47.

Recker, R. 1985. Calcium absorption and achlorhydria. *New England Journal of Medicine* 313:70–73.

Reid, I. R. 1994. Benefits, risks and costs of calcium supplementation in postmenopausal women. *Pharmacoeconomics* 5(1):1–4.

Rosen, C. J. 1994. Premature graying of the hair is a risk factor for osteopenia. *The Journal of Endocrinology and Metabolism* 79(3):854–857.

Rude, R. K. and M. Olerich. 1996. Magnesium deficiency: Possible role in osteoporosis associated with gluten-sensitive enteropathy. *Osteoporosis International* 6:453–61.

Scarbeck, K. 1995. Strength training may reduce the risk of osteoporotic fractures. *Family Practice News* February 15:10.

Scientific Advisory Board, Osteoporosis Society of Canada. 1996. Clinical practice guidelines for the diagnosis and management of osteoporosis. *Canadian Medical Association Journal* 155(8):1113–33.

Seeman, E. 1997. Osteoporosis: Trials and tribulations. *American Journal of Medicine* 103(2A):74S–87S; discussion 87S–89S.

Siani, A. and P. Strazzullo. 1996. Why and how to increase dietary potassium intake. *Nutrition, Metabolism, and Cardiovascular Disease* 6:245–54.

Slemenda, C. 1997. Prevention of hip fractures: Risk-factor modification. *American Journal of Medicine* 103(2A):65S–71S

Teesalu, S. et al. 1996. Nutrition in prevention of osteoporosis. *Scandinavian Journal of Rheumatology* 25(Suppl. 103):81–82.

Weimer, J. P. 1997. Many elderly at nutritional risk. *Nutrition Week* 27(34):4–6.

Werbach, M. R. 1988. *Nutritional Influences on Illness.* Tarzana, CA: Third Line Press.

Wyshak, G. and R. Frisch. 1994. Carbonated beverages, dietary calcium, the dietary calcium/phosphorous ratio, and bone fractures in girls and boys. *Journal of Adolescent Health* 15:210–15.

INDEX